Community
Health Narratives

Community Health Narratives

A Reader

Edited by
EMILY MENDENHALL
and ### KATHY WOLLNER

Foreword by BECHARA CHOUCAIR
Illustrations by HANNAH ADAMS BURQUE

UNIVERSITY OF NEW MEXICO PRESS | ALBUQUERQUE

© 2015 by the University of New Mexico Press
All rights reserved. Published 2015
Printed in the United States of America
20 19 18 17 16 15   1 2 3 4 5 6

Library of Congress Cataloging-in-Publication Data
Community health narratives : a reader / edited by Emily Mendenhall and Kathy Wollner ;
foreword by Chicago Commissioner of Public Health, Bechara Choucair ; illustrations by
Hannah Adams Burque.
    pages cm
 Includes index.
 ISBN 978-0-8263-5559-1 (pbk. : alk. paper) — ISBN 978-0-8263-5560-7 (electronic)
  1. Community health services—Cross-cultural studies. 2. Public health—Cross-cultural studies.
 3. Medical care—Cross-cultural studies. I. Mendenhall, Emily, 1982– editor. II. Wollner, Kathy,
 1986– editor. III. Choucair, Bechara, writer of foreword. IV. Burque, Hannah Adams, illustrator.
  RA427.C6165 2015
  362.12—dc23
                2014023115

Cover illustration: Hannah Adams Burque

Contents

Foreword | ix
BECHARA CHOUCAIR

Acknowledgments | xiii

Introduction | 1
EMILY MENDENHALL

Section I: Social Ties 6

1. Seeking SUCCESS | 10
LAUREN SLUBOWSKI KEENAN-DEVLIN

2. The Big Fat Truth | 27
JUDI MARCIN

3. Dadi's Chart | 35
LESLEY JO WEAVER

4. Mai'suka, My Island | 43
KELLEY ALISON SMITH AND CHANDRA Y. OSBORN

5. Thiago and the Beach | 51
BRIAN ACKERMAN

COMMUNITIES IN ACTION
The Gay-Straight Alliance Network | 61
KATHY WOLLNER

Section II: Gender & Sexuality 64

6. Slow Motion | 68
PATRICK KLACZA

7. Nditai's Initiation | 75
FIONA CRESSWELL

8. Chris Not Christina | 80
JUDI MARCIN

9. Ariana's Decision | 88
KATHY WOLLNER

10. My Body, My Self | 101
MOLLY O'BRIEN AND AUNCHALEE E. L. PALMQUIST

COMMUNITIES IN ACTION
Texas Freedom Network | 114
KATHY WOLLNER

Section III: Mental Health 116

11. The Ties That Bind | 120
NEELY MYERS

12. Chantalle's Secret | 133
ASHLEY HAGAMAN

13. A Homecoming | 140
ERIN P. FINLEY

14. Tenzin's Dream | 149
SARA LEWIS

COMMUNITIES IN ACTION
Sangath | 161
KATHY WOLLNER

Section IV: **Violence** 164

15. Paris of the West | 168
EMBER KEIGHLEY

16. We All Fight | 181
CHARLIE SPEICHER

17. Nelson's Soweto | 188
EMILY MENDENHALL

18. The Grove | 196
SUZANNE FARRELL SMITH

COMMUNITIES IN ACTION
Cure Violence | 206
KATHY WOLLNER

Section V: **Prevention** 208

19. Gone Goes the Worm | 212
ADAM KOON

20. A Pandemic Pig Tale | 225
ERICA GIBSON

21. Route 100 | 235
SUZANNE FARRELL SMITH

22. Girl Parts | 246
JUDI MARCIN

COMMUNITIES IN ACTION
Sabin Vaccine Institute | 255
KATHY WOLLNER

Section VI: Health-Care Access 258

23. Scars | 262
STEPHEN LAVENBERG

24. Mandy and the Motorized Wheelchair | 278
PATRICK KLACZA

25. Open Secrets and Breaking Hearts | 283
HEATHER WURTZ

26. There Will Always Be More Struggles to Win | 291
LESLEY JO WEAVER AND DAVID MEEK

COMMUNITIES IN ACTION
BRAC | 299
KATHY WOLLNER

Postscript | 302
EMILY MENDENHALL

Teaching Guide | 305
KATHY WOLLNER

Contributors | 328

Index | 335

Foreword

Bechara Choucair

I grew up during the civil war in Beirut, Lebanon. In the midst of the chaos and strife that comes hand in hand with armed conflict, I was relatively fortunate. My parents did their best to keep our family safe. They worked hard and made sure that my sisters and I had everything we needed. This afforded me an uninterrupted education and regular access to medical care, something that many children during that time in Beirut were not fortunate enough to receive. It wasn't until years later, with the keen hindsight that comes only with experience, that I realized just how fortunate I had been.

All physicians can recall patients they will never forget. During medical school, I saw patients in a health clinic that provided care to Lebanon's poorest of the poor. One particular patient from that clinic is etched into my memory. She was in her mid-fifties, draped from head to toe in traditional Druze garb, with flowing fabrics. I gathered immediately that she had not seen a doctor in some time, or perhaps ever. She was very timid, and my instincts told me that she was there for more than medical care. She was there to tell me something important. But she was uncomfortable talking to me, perhaps because she was unfamiliar with the medical system or rarely spoke to men alone. She had few resources: no health insurance, formal education, or money to live comfortably in Beirut.

Eventually the woman requested a woman accompany us in the room. The woman then began to explain her problem. She nervously whispered that something had been growing from her vagina for over a year. The mass, now approaching six kilos in weight (more than thirteen pounds), made it difficult to walk. This mass, of course, was cancer. Although she had known of this growth more than a year, she had never sought medical care. This may have been because of shame related to the growth or simply because she did not have access to medical care. Unfortunately, due to the obvious advanced state of her cancer and lack of medical care over her lifetime, it proved fatal.

This woman's condition and death had a profound effect on me. If we had caught her cancer earlier, she could have been treated and lived. Unfortunately, many barriers prevented her from seeking and receiving care. This experience caused me to begin to question the role of social and economic barriers to people's health. I often wondered what it would take for a patient to walk into a clinic at the first sign of a problem.

After medical school, I continued my medical training in the United States. I imagined that things would be different from Lebanon. Surely America had made the systemic changes necessary to ensure universal access to health care and the opportunity to live a healthy life. I was surprised to discover that this was not the case.

When I arrived in the United States, I worked with homeless people, a group I had never encountered in Lebanon. Due to different social and family norms in Lebanon, most people find a place to sleep at night. However, homelessness in America was surprising to me, and I found it to be an incredibly compelling challenge. The homeless in America faced many of the same health issues as did the poorest people in my homeland.

I first worked in Houston, Texas. For a while, I felt I was making a difference, but that feeling did not last long. One of my first patients was a middle-aged man who slept under a bridge yet somehow managed daily access to alcohol and drugs. I eventually engaged him, and we developed together a plan to get him back on track. But he never followed up on the plan. We tried other plans and they all failed. I quickly grew frustrated when I saw him face the same problems over and over again. I felt I couldn't improve my patient's social or health problems. I felt I was failing as a physician.

I knew many of my patients' problems extended beyond the clinic and began to see that I could make a bigger impact at a broader level. I needed to become involved in large-scale system changes so women like the Druze woman I met in Lebanon wouldn't wait until it's too late to access care and my patient experiencing homelessness would have a place to stay with regular access to medical care. These lessons are at the heart of my commitment to community health. Therefore, when I moved to Illinois I shifted my work from individual medical care in the clinic to public health, which focused on the community and policy change.

In 2010, Mayor Richard M. Daley asked me to be the commissioner of the Chicago Department of Public Health. I jumped at this opportunity as I believed that through policy we could make a measureable difference in the health of the people of Chicago, the third largest city in the United States. A year later, along with the newly elected mayor, Rahm Emanuel, I released Healthy Chicago, the first comprehensive public health agenda for our city. The initiative laid out strategies for addressing twelve public health priorities, including obesity, tobacco, HIV prevention, and heart health. This agenda was ambitious because we hoped to make Chicago the healthiest city in the nation.

Since then, we have achieved many goals, from installing healthy vending machines in schools to creating more smoke-free spaces across the city, from more protected bike lanes to low-cost fresh vegetable carts. While individual behavior is important, it's a lot more important for us to change the way our city behaves. With more bike lanes, food-access opportunities, and breastfeeding-friendly hospitals—and with less junk food, tobacco, and unintended pregnancies—I believe we are well on our way to a healthier Chicago.

As commissioner of public health, I've found that awareness of problems is one of the best ways to improve people's health. An individual, group, culture, or society must have the correct information made available to them before any positive outcomes can be achieved. Through reading the stories presented in this book, you will become more aware of public health issues, some common and others shocking, but all realities of the world we live in.

The narratives in this book come from around the world. In some cases, they demonstrate that social problems such as poverty and homelessness can be as real in Beirut as they are in Chicago. But there are also unique challenges that result from certain contexts. As you read this book, you may encounter ideas that are completely foreign to you. I urge you, however, to look for the similarities rather than the differences between the stories and your own life experiences. As you gain awareness, you will be better positioned to make a positive impact in our world.

Bechara Choucair, MD
Commissioner, Chicago Department of Public Health
Follow Dr. Choucair on Twitter: www.twitter.com/choucair

Acknowledgments

The pulse of this book, and other books in this series of health narratives (*Global Health Narratives* and *Environmental Health Narratives*), comes from our contributors, who create stories that engage young readers and encourage them to become curious about public health problems both in their backyard and on the other side of the world. This is the third in a series of books about global publi c health that reaches young readers through narratives. None of the books would be successful without the contributors, their rich experiences working in public health arenas from Texas to Tanzania, and their willingness to share their experiences with us through their stories. We would like to thank those who have contributed to two of the books in the series: Matthew Dudgeon, Leslie Greene, Lauren Slubowski Keenan-Devlin, Brandon A. Kohrt, Adam Koon, Kenneth Maes, Maggie Montgomery, Chandra Y. Osborn, Aunchalee E. L. Palmquist, Ajay Pillarisetti, Jackie Protos, Sarah Raskin, and Suzanne Farrell Smith. We are especially appreciative of Ember Keighley for contributing a story to each of the three books. Thank you for your contributions to this project and your commitment to writing and sharing your knowledge and experience.

The contributors to this book were delightful to work with, and a number of them were exceedingly patient. Some stories were submitted many years ago, and the authors stuck with us as we navigated the waters of book planning and eventually found a home for their contributions. Many contributors have worked extensively in community health endeavors around the globe. Their work as public health practitioners, researchers, teachers, and medical doctors makes this world a better place.

One of the most committed contributors to the Global Health Narratives series is Hannah Adams Burque, our esteemed illustrator. Her commitment and vision is to communicate the series' stories through artwork. This is the third book she has illustrated and we could not be more thankful for her time, creativity, and ability to share a meaningful message.

Finally, we would like to thank our partners, Adam and Patrick, for their ongoing support of this project, through both their written contributions and their enduring encouragement and love as we edited each page of this book. In addition, this book would not have been possible without the many years of love and support from our parents, Barbara and Walter Mendenhall and Pam and Tim Wollner, as we pursued our training and practice in anthropology, medicine, and public health in the classroom, clinic, and community. It is through their examples that we have realized the importance of community in our lives and health as a way to make a small difference in the world.

Introduction

Emily Mendenhall

Mark struggled at school and became depressed because he was bullied.

Sara discovered she was pregnant at fifteen and needed to make a difficult decision about whether to parent.

David suffered from mental illness and learned how to live healthily with it.

Ana Maria feared leaving her home after dark due to gun violence.

Mario and his family benefited from an intervention to prevent the spread of avian flu in his village.

Teresa lacked access to a hospital and was never fully treated.

As defined here, *community health* encompasses many different health issues that affect people living in the same place who generally share similar beliefs and values. In many cases, issues that affect the whole community are very apparent, such as the spread of avian flu, which affected Mario and his family. They benefited from a community-wide intervention to prevent the spread of avian flu. An *intervention* is a project or program that aims to change the course of a health problem. Interventions, which are at the heart of community health, can be used for infectious diseases, such as avian flu, or for other complex health issues, such as obesity. Positive outcomes related to health intervention can be measured in treatment for mental illness, as in David's case, and access to quality health care, which would have allowed Teresa to receive treatment.

However, in other cases, health problems that affect the whole community are less apparent. For example, Mark's struggles, Sara's decision, and Ana Maria's fear may not appear, at first, to be community health issues. But take a closer look. The social relationships we have play an important role in our health, and negative interactions, such as bullying, can have an impact on a person's well-being. The resources provided for young people to make informed decisions and to live healthy lives are also very important. And feeling safe within one's community is an essential part of living a healthy life. These are only some of the issues that may not initially seem like community health issues but require us to recognize that community-level realities can affect people's lives and health in both positive and negative ways.

The definition of community health used in this book includes a broad understanding of the ways in which people, places, and programs shape health. The World Health Organization defines *health* as "a complete state of physical, mental and social well-being, and not merely the absence of disease or infirmity."* However, community health attends to the ways in which the health of a group of people woven together through a common thread—be it a neighborhood, religious institution, school, or tribe—come together to make a whole unit. Therefore, community health is generally measured by disease and suffering at the community level. In public health, this is often measured in how diseases affect morbidity (meaning that a disease affects one's quality of life) and mortality (meaning that someone has died from a disease). Programs and policies are also, therefore, implemented with a focus on communities or collective groups of people.

People are the focus of community health. People also bring the cultural, social, and economic factors of community health into focus. *Culture* describes how people think and behave in relation to a specific group with which they identify; such a group may be one's family,

---

* Preamble to the Constitution of the World Health Organization as adopted by the International Health Conference, New York, June 19–22, 1946, and signed on July 22, 1946, by the representatives of sixty-one states and entered into force on April 7, 1948. World Health Organization, official record 2, Proceedings and Final Acts of the International Health Conference Held in New York from 19 June to 22 July 1946 (June 1948), 100.

friends, or even an institution, such as a school. For example, two common cultural practices in the United States are to gather with family to celebrate Thanksgiving and to exclaim "Bless you" after someone sneezes. We use the term *social* to describe how people interact with others within a prescribed society or group. This might be a family group, friends, a church, or an after-school program where people feel a part of something bigger. Social interactions are especially important because the relationships people have within their social group can influence how they feel, think, and interact with others. Finally, economic factors such as living in poverty influence people's health. This is because the stress of living with limited resources can contribute to one's exposure to disease or limit one's access to health care. In this book we focus on economic, social, and cultural factors that shape how people acquire disease, understand healthy practices, experience illness, and seek treatment.

Places are also very important to community health because some health problems are relevant in some geographic regions of the world but not others. For example, tropical diseases, such as trachoma, are common in countries near the equator, such as Cameroon in Africa, but are nonexistent in Canada in North America, where the natural and built environments are not suitable for trachoma. Tropical diseases originate from structural factors, such as poor sanitation and hygiene, as well as environmental ones, such as the average temperature that promotes the vector (the disease carrier, a fly in this case) to transmit the disease among people. But health problems, such as mental health and violence, can stem from social and cultural factors that can have an equally detrimental effect on people's health. Experiencing a severely traumatic event—for example, sexual abuse or being held at gunpoint—can contribute to depression, anxiety, or post-traumatic stress disorder (PTSD), which can last for a short time or for many years. Some common symptoms of these diseases include withdrawing from society and holding in negative emotions. These experiences also occur in specific places, such as the home or in the street, and can negatively impact how safe people feel in these surroundings. Inherently, these are community issues and need to be addressed as important health concerns that can be transformed by understanding the problem, addressing the problem, and changing how people contribute to it in a certain place and time. Often there are many factors that contribute to problems such as gun violence, and community-wide awareness can make a big impact on reducing it.

Programs are major vehicles for mitigating health problems at the community level. In many cases, public health professionals call these interventions because they are programs whose aim is to change behavior and/or the transmission of a disease in order to improve people's health. In some cases, these programs are developed and carried out by hospitals, but they can also come from grassroots organizations, private voluntary groups, governmental agencies, and after-school programs that function to design, implement, manage, and evaluate community-based public health initiatives. In many cases, people work in their own communities, those neighborhoods or towns where they grew up and maintain relationships, and in other cases, people work to improve community health in communities that are not their own. In both cases, it is important to understand that many factors can influence the success or failure of a public health program. The most important factors are that people in a community believe a health problem affects them and that they want change through the proposed intervention. If people do not identify a health problem as affecting them, although epidemiologists may have identified the problem, it is less likely that an intervention will be successful. Therefore, improvements must come from the bottom up, and people must work together to better the health of their families, friends, and communities.

The narratives in this book, depicting different communities and customs in rich detail, focus on common social and cultural factors that shape community health. They emphasize both individual experiences and how health may be experienced or affected at the community level. In doing so, they explore a wide range of topics: social ties, gender and sexuality, mental illness, violence, prevention, and health-care access. Each of the stories in these topic sections have descriptive introductions addressing each community health topic, providing information on how each issue can be understood and transformed at the community level. "Communities in Action" sketches conclude each section and describe organizations that epitomize good community health programming on the section topic. At the end of the book we provide a teaching guide for teachers who wish to use the book in their classrooms. We suggest using the guide to determine which stories best compliment standard curricula, how to incorporate stories or entire sections into more open-ended curricula, and how to use the community health narratives on their own as a stand-alone education tool.

This book also might be used as a companion to the first two books on global health. While this collection provides some examples from around the world, the majority of its narratives are rooted in the United States. In contrast, *Global Health Narratives: A Reader for Youth* provides a very broad survey of global public health, both thematically and geographically. *Environmental Health Narratives: A Reader for Youth* also surveys the many ways in which the environment can have an impact on people's health, at the individual, community, and even national level. Because the first two books provide such broad examinations of health issues, many stories from those volumes can be used to complement the ones in this book. While this book certainly can be used on its own to discuss fundamental aspects of what makes communities healthy, the three books together provide a comprehensive curriculum that examines people's health experiences across cultures and nations.

This book is a guide to learning about various factors that shape what makes communities healthy and what issues can contribute to poor health in communities in the United States and around the world. By providing these narratives, we aim to enhance young people's understanding of community health, from rural to urban regions and from domestic to global perspectives. Please refer to additional educational resources on our website (Global Health Narratives for Change, www.ghn4c.org).

Section I

Social Ties

The communities we live in and people who surround us influence our health. This section focuses on social ties, which are the relationships we have with family members, friends, neighbors, members of groups (such as at church or school), and even acquaintances. Social ties influence where we live, where and how we learn, what we do for work, what we eat, how we spend our time, and the types of experiences we encounter every day. These relationships can have a major impact on a person's well-being, both mentally and physically. In fact, even having one close friend, relative, or companion you feel understands you can have a direct impact on your health. In contrast, a negative relationship, or a series of difficult social and interpersonal situations, can have a very negative effect on a person's health. Therefore, social ties can affect people's ability not only to cope with disease but also to maintain a healthy life.

Our world is very different from the world of previous generations, and the changes in our world, such as advances in technology, have transformed our social ties. Interactions move at a fast pace, exchanging ideas in minutes, even seconds. Instead of pen pals, which were common among past generations, many people connect through social networking sites like Facebook and Twitter. While in some ways the Internet allows us to be closer to people with whom we wouldn't otherwise be able to communicate, it also means we may be spending more time with technology than building in-person relationships. It is important to recognize the social ties that we build—and how we build them—in our everyday lives.

Most of us try to spend time with people who share common interests, hobbies, or goals and enrich our lives in some way. It's easy to forget that in fact these relationships can profoundly influence our health, as they affect our happiness, our self-esteem, and the choices we make. While the support of one or more friends can affect our health, so can a formalized social network. For example, Alcoholics Anonymous succeeds in helping people stay sober from alcohol because it provides social support to individuals trying to live sober lives. This goes for food choices and exercise routines as well. Eating behaviors play a major role in how healthy you are because if you overeat or eat unhealthy foods, you can become overweight, which can create many long-lasting challenges for your health. Where and with whom you eat can also influence your health. Spending time eating slowly and enjoying healthy foods can improve not only your nutrition but also your emotional well-being.

Social ties are very important for people with chronic illness. Being left alone to care for a disease can be very isolating, but having someone support you, to help you take your medicines, attend health-care appointments, and maintain a healthy lifestyle, can be fundamental to living a healthy life. This support person might be a family member or friend, but it also could be a teacher or social worker. In some cases, young people might fill this role for a parent or grandparent. This can be especially important if the family member does not speak the same language as the health-care provider as a young person might be able to communicate important health information in settings where a formal interpreter is not readily available.

But some social relationships can have a negative impact on an individual's health. For example, when someone decides to quit smoking, one of the most common challenges is to avoid spending time with other people who smoke. We develop relationships around our shared behaviors, and because our friends are often likely to behave as we do, changing one's behavior without breaking social ties can be a struggle. The difficulty of breaking away from unhealthy relationships is one reason why changing behaviors such as overeating or substance use can be a very long, challenging process.

This section describes the ways in which social ties influence health, from eating and activity patterns to emotional well-being and disease management. The section begins with "Seeking SUCCESS," a story that demonstrates the complex ways a difficult home situation and an under-resourced school can affect a young girl's education and a family's health. "The Big Fat Truth" illustrates how bullying can affect one's emotions, self-esteem, and health through direct and indirect ways. In "Dadi's

Chart," Anjali helps her grandmother manage her diabetes by believing in her ability to make the changes her doctor recommends for her. "Mai'suka, My Island" describes how social relationships can have a negative impact on health and illustrates the important role of community-level interventions for behavior changes. Finally, "Thiago and the Beach" demonstrates how a strong friendship can have a positive impact on a person's well-being.

As you read through this section, think about the following questions:

- Are there people in your life who have a positive or negative impact on your health? How so?
- Can you transform a relationship from a difficult to a positive one? How might you do that, and what positive change could it bring to your life?
- If you have or were to have a chronic illness, who is or would be the person you depend upon? Do you play the role of the support person to a family member or friend?

1

Seeking SUCCESS

Lauren Slubowski Keenan-Devlin

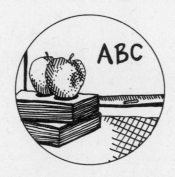

"Seeking SUCCESS*" highlights how family and teachers can limit or transform young people's lives and ultimately their health. Taylor is a ten-year-old girl growing up in a low-income urban neighborhood in the United States. Her mother and father use drugs and alcohol, and her grandmother has cancer. Additionally, Taylor is struggling in school. Like many children growing up in poor city neighborhoods, Taylor attends a school that has too many students and too few resources. She has not learned to read by the fourth grade, and she may be held back. Children like Taylor are at high risk for dropping out of school before graduation and are often trapped in a cycle of poverty because they cannot land a high-paying job without a high school diploma. Differences in access to education or quality of education are a huge driver of racial differences in health outcomes and illuminate the need for better educational and social support services in neighborhoods like Taylor's.*

Taylor gently patted her grandmother's arm before she swung her backpack over one shoulder. "Have a good appointment today, Maw Maw. I love you."

The old woman strained to nod at her granddaughter. The cancer seemed to be causing her a lot of pain today. It had already claimed her breast and was now spreading through her bones. She was only sixty-three but looked a lifetime older.

Taylor glanced at her tiny brother as she walked out the door. At four years old, he was a handful for Maw Maw—she wished her mother would stay off drugs long enough to see that. It was her mother's fault that Maw Maw was falling apart. Maw Maw spent so much time picking up the pieces from her daughter's mistakes that she didn't have the time to go to the doctor when the pain began, when her breast started turning purple and puckered from the tumor. Maybe if she hadn't been so run down from all of the worry that her junkie daughter had caused her, the cancer would never have started.

With a slam of the door, Taylor set off down the sidewalk toward Horatio Elementary. A gust of wind caused the candy wrappers, chip bags, and crushed soda bottles that littered the sidewalk to dance across her path. If she closed her eyes, she could imagine them as fallen leaves crunching beneath her feet.

Taylor slid into her seat just as the school bell rang. Slumping down low and propping her feet on the back of the desk in front of her, she heaved a sigh and let her mind wander, as usual, far away from the classroom. Today Taylor thought about her grandmother and was only reminded of Ms. Hamlin's presence when the teacher's voice sharpened to call order to the unruly, overcrowded classroom. Ms. Hamlin scratched letters on the board, but to Taylor they were nonsense; she had never learned to read properly. Books and worksheets looked like word-search puzzles. She didn't even bother to put her homework in her backpack these days, since her time at home was spent watching her brother, Little Man, so Maw Maw could rest. Rest. That sounded nice right about now. Taylor let her heavy eyelids droop closed.

"Markus, go to the disciplinarian's office!" Ms. Hamlin bellowed.

Taylor's eyes popped open. "Now, it's time for science. Get out your books. Princess, put the phone away or it's mine!"

Taylor adjusted herself in her seat and switched her pencil between hands, staring out the window in preparation for the next lesson.

"Who can tell me what a 'hypothesis' is?" asked Ms. Hamlin. A girl at the front of the classroom answered. "Right," Ms. Hamlin said, "so it's an idea that you think is right. For example, I could say, my hypothesis is 'only people with bad behaviors, like people who smoke, get cancer.'"

Taylor jolted in her seat. "That's not true!" she cried, now sharply tuned in.

"Don't yell out in my class, Taylor!" warned Ms. Hamlin. "That's my hypothesis. Now how could I go about testing this hypothesis?"

"It's a stupid hypothesis!" hollered Taylor, her face burning with rage.

"That's enough! Taylor, go join Markus in the disciplinarian's office," said Ms. Hamlin.

"I don't care if you're the teacher," Taylor mumbled under her breath as she rose from her seat, eyes fixed on her instructor's outstretched arm and pointed finger. "You don't know what you're talking about." Dragging her backpack by one strap, Taylor stormed angrily out of the room.

Taylor couldn't wait to get home to check on Maw Maw. Scurrying up the path, she found the front door wide open, but her grandmother wasn't in her easy chair. Instead, she found her mother in the bedroom dumping armfuls of clothing into boxes.

"What's going on, Mom?"

"Maw Maw's dying. She went in for a checkup, and they won't let her leave, darn hospital. You kids got to go to your dad's house."

Taylor's stomach dropped. "For how long?"

"We ain't coming back here, OK? Even if she comes home by some miracle, she can't watch Little Man. What the heck am I supposed to do with him?" Her mother shoved her frail frame against the top of an over-filled box, attempting to close it with a force she didn't have. "Be useful! Go feed your brother or help me pack."

Taylor was never allowed to be emotional—crying got you beat, and it never solved anything, anyway. Sturdily, Taylor walked out into the living room where Little Man sat on the floor, staring at the television. "Ya hungry, Little Man?"

Her dad was propped on the couch, feet on the coffee table, surrounded by discarded beer cans when the family of three dragged their boxes through the front door that night. "Hey, kids," he offered, obviously buzzed from his drinks. There were a few other adults in the room as well, all in similar states of drunkenness. "Y'all are in the downstairs room. Tay Tay, leave Little Man with us and take your things down there."

"Yeah, you do that, Tay Tay," echoed her mother, dropping a half-opened box on the floor. "I'm going out."

The next morning, Taylor woke with the sun glinting through the basement glass block window. It took her forever to find a clock in the house. She finally spotted one on the crusty oven in the basement kitchen and saw she was already ten minutes late for school. Taylor threw on her uniform, sweeping her short, textured hair under a beanie cap, and headed upstairs. Little Man was asleep on the sofa next to his father. A couple of the other adults were still in place, too, heads rolled back, breathing loudly. Her father was not very reliable, but he was more reliable than her mother. Taylor knew Little Man would still be alive when she came home, so she forced herself out the door and down the sidewalk toward Horatio School.

At least her father's block was better than Maw Maw's. Just around the corner were a candy store, a good fast-food restaurant, and a corner store. Not even a block away, Taylor passed by the gated front door of Kid Korner, an after-school program that a lot of her classmates attended. She was already late, so she slowed just a bit to look up at the sign. The dot over the *i* in "Kid" was shaped like a flying basketball, zooming toward the rim and net that formed the *o* in "Korner." Taylor yearned to play basketball at school, but the school could barely afford text books, let alone a gym or sports equipment. Maybe Kid Korner would let her play, now that she lived around the block. Taylor made a mental note to herself as she picked up speed, hustling to beat the second bell that would mean detention.

Taylor didn't stop to talk to anyone after school that day—she had to get back home to ask her dad about Kid Korner. Today she found him in the yard, hanging over the fence and talking to a neighbor as Little Man kicked around the dirt and weeds.

"Hey, Dad? Could I go to that place around the block—you know, Kid Korner? Could I go today?"

Her dad shrugged. "Sure, I don't see why not!" he hollered loudly. "Take your brother too. I got people coming."

Taylor knelt down to talk to Little Man. "Come on, I think this could be fun," she told her brother tenderly as she took his hand. Little Man was painfully shy, but he went wherever his sister took him. The two turned back up the block to make the short walk to Kid Korner.

At 3:45 p.m., the front door looked much friendlier than it had that morning. The gate was pushed aside, and the bright-green door reflected the afternoon sunlight. Nervous and hopeful, Taylor reached up to ring the big black doorbell mounted on the brick building.

A moment later, the door swung inward. A large, bearded man appeared in the doorway, his eyes drawn narrow. His deep, booming voice was startling. "And who are you?"

"Uh, my name is Taylor, I go by Tay Tay. This is my little brother, Ray. We call him 'Little Man.' We was wondering if we can come in."

The narrow eyes narrowed even more, and the bearded face hung in the doorway for another moment before ushering the two kids inside.

As Little Man clung tightly to her side, Taylor shuffled past the man into a small vestibule lined with old couches and mismatched chairs. Hundreds of young, dark faces stared down from the walls: smiling images of neighborhood children, playing and posing, sporting clothing and hairstyles from the past several decades.

"You know some of these kids?" His voice came much more softly now.

Taylor nodded. "I go to school with Kennelly and Ruby. And that looks like my big cousin Tavarion, but he's grown now."

"That's Tavarion, all right. That picture's gotta be ten years old," said the man.

Lowering his large frame into an overstuffed green couch, the man let out a slight grunt. "I'm Dan, Tay Tay. And how old is this guy?" he asked, glancing down at Little Man.

Taylor felt a wave of nerves. She didn't know much about this place, but she didn't think they let little kids come if they weren't in school yet. "Uh, five?"

Dan now looked down at Little Man. "How old are you, Little Man?"

The scared child held up four tiny fingers then buried his face in Taylor's arm.

"Oh, so he's five, is he?" chuckled Dan, imitating Little Man's gesture. He shook his head. "Is there someone at home to watch him? He's really too young for us."

Taylor's face hardened now. She thought about Little Man playing with beer cans, surrounded by cigarette smoke as his father played cards with his buddies late into the night. "No, there's no one to watch him."

Dan looked Taylor squarely in the eye, as though trying to read her thoughts. After several moments, his gaze softened, a look of understanding coming into his eyes. "OK. Here's the deal. He can stay, but he's your responsibility. He's with you, all the time. Is that clear?"

Taylor felt a wave of relief. "OK, thank you," she said gratefully.

"Go on in the cafeteria and get a snack, one for each of you. We start at three thirty every day, so make sure you're on time tomorrow. Now, go on!"

The two shuffled into the cafeteria, and Taylor scanned the room full of faces. She knew at least half of the twenty kids in the room, many of whom called to her or waved. Her friend Ruby hopped up from a table and ran over to hug her. Dan walked in the room and shouted, "Free time!" and the crowd responded by leaping up from their tables and scurrying off to other rooms in the building. Taylor followed Ruby and a small group of kids through a big, open space and into a small concrete room with boarded-up windows, exposed pipes, and a worn-out basketball rim attached to a plywood backboard. With Little Man waiting quietly in the corner, Taylor and the older kids played game after game of knockout, horse, and three-on-three. If there was a heaven, Taylor thought, this was close to it.

But her high came crashing down when, an hour later, one of the teenage counselors stuck her head in the door and bellowed, "Homework time! Go to your rooms!"

The counselor pointed to Taylor. "Take your last shot—you're with me. Let's go." Sharing a chair with Little Man at a big round table in a tiny, windowless room, Taylor watched her Kid Korner peers take out their schoolbags and remove folders, books, and worksheets.

"Hi, Tay Tay, I'm Brittany. You got your homework?"

Taylor shook her head. "We didn't get no homework today."

"Really? OK. Well don't worry about that, we got plenty of stuff here for you to work on. What kind of math are you doing in school?"

Taylor smiled. You didn't have to be a good reader to be good at math. Brittany dug through a bin of papers and pulled out several multiplication worksheets. Taylor spent the next hour whizzing through worksheet after worksheet. Homework time didn't seem so bad after all.

Every day that week, Taylor and Little Man made their way to Kid Korner. It was a welcome relief from the chaos of home: unknown adults in and out every day, a drunken father uninterested in how late his small kids stayed out, and a mother always on the verge of going to jail for her heroin habit. Pounding the ball against the pavement of the basketball room at Kid Korner also helped Taylor to keep her mind off of her sick grandmother, whom she visited every weekend at the nursing home. Taylor could breathe here, relax here.

The following Monday, Taylor could hardly wait to get back to Kid Korner. The door swung open, predictably, at 3:30, and Taylor flew through the entryway, nearly colliding with one of the counselors. Looking up, she saw Brittany with her fists on her hips, lips pursed, and brow furrowed.

"Let me guess, no homework for you today, right?"

Taylor hesitantly began to shake her head.

"That's funny," said Brittany, her right thumb jabbing over her shoulder toward no one in particular, "because Kayvon is in your class, and he told me you had loads of homework last week, and a whole packet for today."

Taylor stood there with her mouth open, wanting to defend herself but without a word in her head.

"Leave Little Man here with Dan, he'll be fine." Brittany thrust her hand out in front of her, palm up. "You and me got business. Let's go, Tay Tay."

Hand in hand, the two marched down the street to the elementary school, right into the principal's office. Mrs. Madison sat behind her desk, waiting expectantly, an open folder filled with papers in front of her.

"Thanks for meeting with us, Mrs. Madison. I called the school last Friday to see why Taylor hasn't been getting any homework, and I found out that she hasn't turned in an assignment all semester. Her teacher said she's failing. I wanted to see what we can do about it."

Mrs. Madison pulled out a piece of paper and placed it atop the file. "Yes, I'm afraid Taylor's going to have to repeat the fourth grade at this point." The principal proceeded to show Brittany progress reports littered with Fs and Ds as well as sample tests that Taylor had left mostly blank. "She comes late most of the days she's here and has missed so many days of school that she's better off just doing this year over again."

Brittany's face was a mix of shock, disappointment, and anger. "How will she be better off? How can you guarantee that she'll pass it the second time through? Why didn't anybody do anything to help her earlier?"

The principal let out a pointed sigh. "Look, miss, I have 560 other kids to worry about in this school. We've been on academic probation for the past seven years, but they're not giving us any extra supplies, money, or teachers to make things any better. Taylor's instructor has thirty-two other kids in her room. My one-on-one teaching aids are all working with the students who can't walk through the hallways without punching someone or damaging school property. We just can't do everything here. What other choice do I have but to hold her back?"

Brittany's face was soft now, her voice gentle. "Let me help," she offered. "Tay Tay comes to our program every day. I'll work with her for the rest of the school year, and all through summer school. If she can get As and Bs for the rest of her assignments, can you pass her in the fall?"

"Happily," said Mrs. Madison without pause.

Back at Kid Korner, the two set to work. Taylor's problem quickly became apparent to Brittany, as Taylor struggled to read the instructions on her science worksheet. The girl had never learned to read but had somehow been passed through kindergarten, first grade, second, and third.

"Why didn't you say something to me, to anyone?" asked Brittany.

Taylor lowered her eyes. "I tried. I told my second-grade teacher that I didn't get it, but she never had time to help me. And Maw Maw can barely see. And my mom is never around. They all just told me to learn at school. After a while, I just gave up."

Brittany shook her head. "Well, better late than never. Let me get the sight-word flash cards. We'll start there."

✸

The pair worked during every spare minute of the day through June, July, and August. Once Taylor had mastered reading, the challenges of home-work seemed to melt away. Science, social studies, and vocabulary made a lot more sense when she could actually understand the directions. At the end of August, Brittany and Taylor met for a second time with Mrs. Madison.

"I am so proud of you, Taylor," the principal said, beaming. "And thank you for all of your help, Brittany. Taylor went from failing fourth grade to earning all As and two Bs in summer school. What excellent progress! Her teacher said she's even paying more attention in class, now that she can see the board with the new glasses she got through Kid Korner. Taylor, I am happy to pass you on to fifth grade."

✸

Things were looking way, way up for Taylor. Besides her own achieve-ments with Kid Korner and passing school, Maw Maw was finally returning home from the nursing home. While the cancer hadn't gone away, the doctors had found medicines that helped her feel comfortable. Taylor couldn't wait to visit on Saturday and tell Maw Maw the great news about school.

The old woman looked rested, sitting in her favorite recliner with her hair freshly washed. Taylor hugged her gently and sat on the end of the neighboring couch.

"We missed you, Maw Maw," she said earnestly.

"You too, baby. It's good to be home." Grunting slightly as she shifted her weight, Maw Maw reached over to the end table and picked up five small plastic canisters. "Do me a favor, Tay, and read these bottles for me. I got to take these at different times, and I'll be darned if I can remember which."

A few months earlier, Taylor's heart would have sunk in her chest at such a request. But now she felt proud to be able to help her grandmother. "This one you need to take in the afternoon, with food. Wanna take it with some crackers now?"

Maw Maw nodded, and Taylor grabbed the box from the kitchen shelf. "Say, what if I lay out all of your pills in the kitchen, in little cups or something, so you don't have to try to read the bottles every day? Would you like that?"

"Bless you, child!" her grandmother smiled. "I'm lucky you're so smart."

And for the first time, Taylor felt smart too.

At Kid Korner the following Monday, Taylor spent all her free time in the computer lab, slowly pecking at the keyboard with two fingers. "How do you get cancer?" she typed into the search window, scrolling through the options on the screen.

"Too much sunlight causes skin cancer," noted one website.

"Exposure to toxic chemicals can cause various cancers," stated another.

She printed off page after page of information from various websites, securing the papers with several staples and a paper clip. "Good people get cancer too," she wrote across the top of the first page. The next day, she walked up to school, buzzed into the front office, and slipped the packet of papers into Ms. Hamlin's mailbox. "Told you that was stupid," she said, smiling as she skipped back down the front stairs.

As September breezes cooled off the scorching summer sun, the schoolchildren made their way back to Horatio Elementary. This year, Taylor didn't dread the four-block walk nearly as much. Brittany's support and confidence over the summer reassured her, as did the tiny company with whom she walked hand in hand: Little Man had turned five in July and was beginning kindergarten this year.

Walking into her classroom on this first day of school, Taylor held her head a little higher than last year. She took a seat a bit closer to the board and sat up a little straighter. When the teacher asked her to read aloud from her social studies packet, Taylor felt proud that the words came easier and faster, and Mrs. Haversy praised her loudly when she finished.

But as the days turned to weeks, and the weeks to months, an unfamiliar emotion started bubbling up inside her. In the past, Taylor spaced out during lessons or spent her time doodling on the desk, but now she paid more attention to the classroom around her. And things in here moved slowly. Mrs. Haversy spent at least ten minutes in the beginning of class just trying to settle down the students. When it was Taylor's peers' turn to answer a question or write on the board, Taylor's mind raced ahead, waiting anxiously for her classmates to catch up. In-class reading sessions were agonizing.

At the end of January, Mrs. Haversy handed out progress reports. Not bothering to open the envelope, Taylor tucked it into her pocket and headed out into the icy wind to make her way to Kid Korner.

"Have something for me, Tay?" asked Dan as she walked in the building.

Taylor nodded, pulling the crushed envelope from her jacket. Dan quickly unfolded the form.

Within a moment, his face crumpled into a deep frown. "Tay Tay! What are these grades about? A C in reading and a C in social science? That's not you! What's going on?"

Taylor was a bit surprised herself. She gave Dan a puzzled shrug.

"Don't you shrug at me!" he bellowed. Taylor jumped—she had rarely seen Dan so angry, and never with her before. Swinging abruptly out of his seat, Dan barked, "Come with me!" and stormed into his office. Taylor followed timidly.

More gently now, as she closed the office door, Dan prodded Taylor for an answer. "You are way too bright to be getting grades like this. You made honor roll last semester. What happened?"

"I don't know," said Taylor meekly. "I guess . . . I guess I been bored in class. The other kids are just so slow! And the homework's too easy. I guess that's why I not been doing it. I just keep telling Brittany I done it already."

Dan was no longer angry. "So you're not feeling challenged anymore. Well, that's something we can fix. You need to come talk to me about these things, or come to Brittany. That's what we're here for. Got it?"

Taylor nodded.

"Now, I think I might have a solution. Let me make a couple of phone calls."

❖

Two weeks later, on Saturday, Dan called home to speak with Taylor's dad. Taylor's father listened carefully, nodded along, mumbled agreement, and finally hung up after ten minutes. "Hey Tay," he coughed, clearing his throat. "Dan wants you at Kid Korner. He says come in an hour and put on your school uniform. He got someone there for you to meet or somethin'."

Taylor wasn't sure what to expect as she pushed that familiar doorbell. The door swung open, and Dan's hairy face appeared in the dark opening. "The SUCCESS folks just got here. They're excited to meet you! Remember what we talked about, OK? Just relax, and be yourself."

Following Dan into one of the classrooms, Taylor was bursting with curiosity as she entered the room to find two adults, a black man and a white woman, seated at the large round table. The adults stood and smiled when Taylor entered the room, and the woman extended her hand: "It's nice to meet you, Tay. I'm Ms. McKinley. This is my colleague, Mr. Peters."

"How do you do, Taylor," echoed Mr. Peters. "We're from SUCCESS Academy. We heard from Mr. Dan here about your academic capabilities. We would like to see if you might be a good fit for our school."

The three adults and the fifth grader spent an hour talking about Taylor's family, her recent move, and her time at Kid Korner. Next,

Ms. McKinley and Mr. Peters gave Taylor a series of oral and written tests. Afterward, the four of them chatted some more before the instructors finally stood up and offered their hands once again.

"What a pleasure to get to know you, Taylor," said Ms. McKinley. She glanced at Mr. Peters, who gave a slight nod. "We think you would be a great candidate for SUCCESS Academy. Would you like to come on Monday and spend a day in the classroom to learn more about us?"

Taylor nodded eagerly. "Yes! I'd love that!"

🔲

Taylor rushed out the door that afternoon, turning right instead of her usual left, and practically jogged the six blocks to her grandmother's place.

"Hey, Maw Maw! Guess what!" she hollered, swinging the door shut behind her.

"Hi, Tay," her grandmother answered. "What's got you all excited?"

"I met these great teachers from a new school, Maw Maw! They talked to me and Dan, and they think I should come visit and maybe even start there! It sounds real great. Dan's gonna take me on Monday."

Maw Maw's face lit up. "Aw, Tay, good for you. I always known you was bright. If any of my grandkids gonna go to college, it's you, Tay. I just can't say enough how important school is for your future."

Maw Maw's eyes wandered off as she finished her sentence, fixing in a faraway stare. She was no longer smiling but looked sad and wistful.

"Your momma." She paused. "That girl coulda been somethin', too, you know." Maw Maw shook her head, sighing. "I thought I was doin' right by her, but I didn't teach her like I shoulda. She started messing with an older boy, a gangbanger, when she was fourteen, and I never taught her about taking care of herself. Before I know it, she come home pregnant. I didn't make her study or nothing. I was mad and told her she had to stay home and take care of that baby, your big sister. Without school, she couldn't get no job besides running drugs for that gangbanger boyfriend. She was depressed, and started using drugs, and . . ."

Maw Maw now turned to look at her granddaughter. "Tay, I want better for you. I want you to stick with school. I want you to have a better life, to be healthy, and happy."

Taylor nodded silently. She had never known these things about her mother. But Taylor knew she didn't want to be like that haggard, worn-down woman who came in and out of her life. She was relieved as her thoughts turned back to SUCCESS Academy. This school could be the stroke of luck she needed.

Dan drove Taylor to the school that next Monday. It was a long drive outside of her neighborhood, and she would have to ride on two buses to get there. But Maw Maw's voice was in her head as they pulled up to the front door, and as the day went on, Taylor became more and more convinced that the school was worth the trip. She loved every minute there. She loved the rhymes that the students recited as reminders of SUCCESS's rules and ethics; she loved the clean hallways, shiny textbooks, and friendly teachers; and most of all, she loved the enormous basketball court and the coach who told her, after watching a short scrimmage, that she was a natural.

As Dan dropped Taylor off at her dad's house that evening, he looked her in the eye and heaved a heavy breath. "So, Tay. I know you love it. But the question is, will your father be willing to sign you up?"

"Why wouldn't he? Everything's great there! I'm going to learn so much. I'm going to be 'Happy, Healthy, and SUCCESSful!'" she cried, reciting the school motto.

"Well, adults sometimes have a hard time seeing past themselves. Talk with him and see what he says."

Her dad was sitting in the corner by the television, the flicker of the screen the only light in the dark room. "Tay Tay!" he hollered when he saw her in the doorway. "How's it going?"

Taylor hesitated. "Good, Dad. You remember how I went to SUCCESS today?"

"Huh?" he grunted, his eyes still on the television.

"Dad, I went to that new school today. It was real, real great. I want to go full-time. Can you sign me up?"

Taylor's dad was looking at her now, his face stiff. "Where it at? By your brother's school?"

"Well, no, it's the other way. I got to take the bus. But that's OK, 'cause cousin Tonisha used to stay over there, so I know where I'm going."

Her dad was still expressionless. "What about your brother? Who gonna walk him to school then?"

Taylor wasn't sure how to respond. "Could you walk him?"

"You want me to get up at the crack of dawn every day to walk Little Man to school? What's so special about this place that I gotta do that for you?"

"It's just great, Dad, really. And I'm going to learn so much more, and play basketball on the team!"

Her dad turned his face back to the television. "Nah, Tay, I don't think so. You got a school already. You learn plenty there. I didn't have no fancy school, I don't see why you need one. You don't need to be smarter than your pops. I'm all you need."

Taylor felt like the air had been sucked out of her lungs, as though she'd run straight into a cement wall. Tears welled to the edge of her eyelashes. She never cried, but now she couldn't stop the tears from spilling down her face.

"Please?" she whispered, barely audible.

"I said no, Tay. Now go get your brother, he's over at Jamison's house."

The walk to school that next morning was harder than it had ever been. The cold stabbing at her cheeks was nothing compared to the hollow feeling that filled her insides. Entering the hallways, everyone around her moved in slow motion; the fighting, the yelling, the laughing, and the shouting all felt distant and disconnected.

Taking a seat in the back of the class, Taylor thought about the beginning of the school year. She remembered how happy she had been to be in this classroom, to read and learn, to feel smart. Smart people get to be something, she thought. They finish high school, and some even go to college. She thought of her older cousins, who had all dropped out before finishing high school. They were on the streets now, one using drugs like Taylor's mother and another running stolen goods for his gang. Tonisha was only seventeen and had had two babies already—she could barely get by with her job at Burger King and was constantly moving from place to place, crashing on friends' couches.

Taylor's thoughts turned to Maw Maw. When you're smart, you can make people's lives better, you can take care of yourself and your family. Who would be helpin' Maw Maw if I hadn't learned to read? But this classroom was a trap, just like the rest of her neighborhood. She wasn't going anywhere so long as she was sitting in this crowded, tired room.

Taylor stared out the window, her eyes tracing the line where the rooftops met the sky. It was a stunningly bright shade of blue today. She imagined the view from the windows of SUCCESS Academy, and let out a long, slow breath as she slid down into her seat, propping her feet on the desk in front of her.

The teacher began the long, slow process of quieting her fellow students. And Taylor felt herself slowing down to meet them.

2

The Big Fat Truth

Judi Marcin

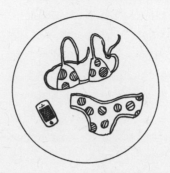

"The Big Fat Truth" tells a story of cyberbullying. Bullying and cyberbullying have become commonplace in American culture, particularly among middle and high school students. Bullying can have major ramifications for the person being bullied, such as negative emotions, embarrassment, and loss of self-esteem, and for the person doing the bullying, such as legal problems. In this story Mel loses her cell phone after a debate and someone posts photos of her on Facebook that she never would have posted herself. This mortifying episode causes her intense grief yet has a hopeful outcome.

Mel sat in the auditorium and waited for the debate-team tryouts. It was the fourth day of school. She tucked her hair behind her ears and fidgeted in her seat. Most things about this place made her fidget: the heat, the bugs, the sandspurs. A month ago she and her mother were in Portland, Oregon. Now they lived in St. Petersburg, Florida. It was not exactly how she planned to spend her sophomore year. Mel yanked at her polo shirt so it didn't cling against her chest and stomach and tugged at her skirt. The mandated uniform was another source of fidgeting and irritation. Required dress was the sworn enemy of any plus-sized, curvy girl. It never leveled the playing field. However, it did show people how much she *didn't* look like everyone else.

The St. Petersburg Academy required a navy plaid skirt and white polo shirt *every day*, which were nothing like the long-sleeved band T-shirts and torn jeans Mel was most comfortable in. What made the polo shirt worse was its whiteness. White made her already noticeable midsection that much more noticeable and it was a magnet for sloshed drinks. More hideous than the skirt and shirt were the knee socks. Mel's thick and sturdy calves shoved into pencil-thin knee-highs were like two giant pythons trying to squeeze through coffee stirrer straws.

Mel was tall like her mother, six foot two. But unlike her mother, a professional beach volleyball player (hence the move to Florida), Mel despised anything athletic and detested every sport she had ever tried. Basketball, volleyball, soccer—all those coaches were sure she was the perfect fit, until she actually played. Within fifteen minutes of tryouts she would hear, "Thanks for coming out. We'll call you if a spot opens up." She knew she was a klutz. She could trip over dirt. It was like her brain and body spoke two different languages. The clumsiness is why she started reading everything she could. And the reading made her more curious. And her curiosity got her on the debate team.

On a debate team, there were no jump shots or spikes, no free throws or free kicks, no goalkeeping. There was a podium, herself, her team-mate, and her opponents. People saw her brain not her body. She battled with words and wit rather than brawn and brute force.

Mel wanted the top spot on the St. Petersburg Academy debate team. She wanted the spot left by the great Charles Radcliffe, the YouTube sensation known for the Radcliffe Method of Debate. His excellence put the St. Petersburg Academy on the debate-world map and earned him a scholarship to Georgetown University. In Portland, Mel had won awards in sectional and regional competitions but found Portlanders a little too laid back when it came to intense competition. Gaining the top spot on the team would compensate for having to wear a school uniform rather than shorts, T-shirts, and sandals in a place that was hotter than the sun.

In proper debate tradition, the coveted top spot on the academy team was given to the winner of that final contest. Over the past three weeks, she had eliminated many other hopefuls. Now it came down to herself and Ethan. Ethan was Charles's brother.

Ethan admitted to Mel that he was not exactly sure why he had to compete against her, but he agreed to the debate for the good of the entire team. Mel expected to work hard during the last few weeks of summer preparing for the debate. What she didn't expect was to actually like Ethan. He never sneered at her body but complimented her logic. For him it was all about exceeding expectations, doing the research, putting in the time. His dedication to debate matched her own. Mel wanted to belong in a place where her size didn't matter. She believed this team could be that place and that she and Ethan could actually become friends. For the first time in a long time, Mel allowed herself to be hopeful.

Normally debates are made up of two-person teams who argue either for or against something. In this instance, Mel was the "against," or negative, and Ethan was the "for," or affirmative. The topic was school uniforms. All of the battles Mel had ever had with her body went into that debate. She showed her off her passion, her research, and her intelligence. But so did Ethan. He was just as passionate, just as prepared, and just as smart. They high-fived each other at the end of the thirty minutes because it was an incredible debate.

When Ms. McCallister announced the winner—"Melanie Evans"—Mel did a fist pump and shook Ethan's hand. The team surrounded her, patted her back, and congratulated her. She tried to get Ethan's attention to explain what an honor it was to compete and how close the results must have been when Ethan stormed off stage. He kicked over a metal folding chair. The sound echoed through the auditorium. Mel's heart broke. She felt as empty as that echo, convinced Ethan would never forgive her.

Mel wiped her tears on the collar of her shirt and quickly left school. When she got home, there was a bowl of baby carrots on the counter and a written message: "How did it go? Can't wait to hear. Call me when you get home. Love, Mom." Mel ate three baby carrots to earn the right to eat what she really wanted, a handful of Oreos. Mel loved food, and her mom loved serving sizes. One-eighth of a frozen pizza, a quarter of a pint of ice cream, half of a bagel, thirteen chocolate candies, one ounce of potato chips: it was dieting by a different name. But for Mel it wasn't just about the junk food, which definitely was good. It was about all kinds of food. The really good stuff—interesting meals, international cuisine, molecular gastronomy that used science to play with food—was all amazing and reminded her life could be full of incredible flavors and adventures. She lived to experience food and all its combinations. While Mel saw a great meal as something to look forward to, her mother saw it as an irritating necessity.

When Mel went to call her mom, she couldn't find her cell phone. She dumped out her backpack, went through her pockets, and retraced her steps. No phone. Then she remembered. In the all the excitement of winning the debate, she had never picked up her phone from the table backstage. Mel walked back to school as fast as she could, and the kind security guard let her in. Mel was convinced he felt sorry for her, being that it was Friday. Her look of anxiety and desperation probably helped too. The truth was, she was anxious and desperate. Her friends were all in Portland. Her phone kept her connected. And with Ethan pissed off, she worried things had changed forever.

For some reason people like Mel are never immediately welcomed into the high school world of the popular. For Mel, being overweight was like having some contagious skin rash. People either looked at her funny or avoided her altogether. Eating for the wrong reasons was not good. Doing anything for the wrong reasons was not good. But Mel knew it was math. She took in more calories than she burned up, pure and simple. It was hard: the thing she loved was bad in excess but a necessity in moderation. She knew there was more to her than her size, but most people didn't take the time to understand that.

When Mel couldn't find her phone, she tried to quiet her swells of panic. Certainly no one at the school desperately wanted a three-models-old smart phone when they had the newest tech gadgets any regular teenager would covet. She believed by Monday morning her phone would be returned and all would be right with the world. But on her walk back home, she remembered the pictures.

In a moment of distress, soon after Mel had accepted they were moving to Florida, she took some pictures. Convinced there was no way she could live in Florida if she were overweight, she planned to enter a "before and after" contest. It was part of some weight-loss infomercial. One Saturday morning, she went into a store in downtown Portland and tried on every kind of bathing suit she could find. She took selfies for the "before" shot.

Twenty different kinds of bathing suits and nearly as many pictures later, she looked in the mirror and knew the whole thing was ridiculous. What she would need to sacrifice to make herself look like some of those "after" shots would never be permanent. She liked food too much and had more respect for herself than that. It was OK if she was not a size 2 or 4 or 6, or 12 for that matter. She was never going to be magically transformed. She had to work to find balance, not live for extremes.

Mel's very quick walk became a jog. Winded, she leaned over, hands on her knees, and waited for the "gonna vomit" feeling to pass—not from the running but from the fear that anyone was looking at those pictures. She logged into Facebook with her laptop and nearly choked on another baby carrot.

There, on her timeline, her best friend Jen posted, "You've been hacked." Mel scrolled down and saw fourteen pictures of herself in too-small bathing suits sporting too many skin folds. All the photos had captions:

"Like—your favorite walrus pose."
"Behold the orca."
"Beach time for baby elephant."
"Hungry hungry hippo."
"Ughhh—makes me not so hungry."

There were hateful and hurtful comments from people Mel didn't know, even some whose names she had never heard.

Then she saw the friend-request notifications. Whoever had taken her phone had sent friend requests to everyone on the debate team from her Facebook account. And those people were so well connected to rest of the academy that what started off as nine friend requests became who-knows-how-many views. Mel's breath caught in her chest. Sobs stuck in her throat. She was silent. Her self-worth, her confidence, her identity crumbled inside. She stared at the screen. She had to make a choice. Either she faced this or she hid. Mel was not good at hiding.

The debater and problem-solver side of her took over. In every debate there was a rebuttal. She called Jen.

"Jen, help! What do I do?"

"Give me your password. I'll delete your whole account. We've got to reset everything so whoever's doing this can't keep posting stuff. Do you know how this happened?"

"My phone. Someone stole my phone after debate tryouts."

"Good thing you're picky about Facebook friends and a creature of habit. I knew something had to be up when I saw pics of you rather than your favorite new seafood place. I mean, those comments. Good grief, you have some ruthless people at that new school of yours."

Mel tried to stifle her sobs. "I don't even know those people, but they obviously feel in cyberspace it's completely OK to say horrible things about me."

Jen sighed. "I'm so sorry, Mel. Babe, give me a few and I'll call you back. OK?"

Mel nodded, which of course Jen couldn't hear, so she squeaked out an "OK."

After Mel hung up, she ran through the list of suspects. Ethan popped into her head and Mel tried to push the idea away. He was pissed and he had gone backstage. He lost to the new girl, the fat girl. Maybe he wanted to show everyone just how fat she was. Mel couldn't stop her tears. He had done it with her help, no Photoshop, no fake heads on bodies. Mel cried aloud, "Stupid ideas, stupid, ugly body, and those stupid, stupid, ugly pictures." She flopped her head down on the counter and wondered if her own body could smother itself.

Jen called back. She had reset everything and Mel had a new Facebook account. Jen immediately began to fill it with fun. She posted Mel's favorite food places, best memories, and favorite bands. Mel felt better but knew it wasn't real. Because Monday morning loomed in front of her and she would have to relive the worst hours of her life all over again, this time in front of the entire school.

Mel's mom was away at a volleyball tournament in Miami all weekend, so she didn't tell her anything. Mel spent the weekend watching a John Hughes film marathon, since she owned every one of his movies. She watched *The Breakfast Club* six times and bawled hysterically each time it ended. Mel was sure her own story would not end in Hollywood fashion. Jen called her at least eight times, along with Jack and Min, Lydia and Sean. They wanted to shield her with their love and friendship, but Mel was still the one who had to walk into school alone with nothing but those big fat pictures that showed off the big fat truth.

Mel made sure she was fake asleep when her mom came home on Sunday night. Her mom came into her room, smoothed Mel's hair, and kissed her cheek. She smelled of beach and suntan lotion and hair gel.

When Monday morning arrived, Mel decided to wait until the last possible moment to go to school. That way, she thought, the halls would be empty. But no such luck. Ethan stood near her locker and held out her phone.

"I think this is yours."

She thought of a hundred curses she wanted to yell, but all she said was, "How could you?"

"Wait, what?" He waved his hands out in front of him. "No, no. It wasn't me. It was Ryan, the guy who didn't make the team. He has so few brain cells that not only did he do something that would get him suspended, he went on to brag about it to everyone. I found out and got your phone back."

She wanted to believe him.

"Don't worry. Ryan's not just suspended, he got kicked out—since he stole your phone. Stealing at the academy is immediate dismissal so . . ."

Mel stopped him midsentence and hugged him. Without hesitation he hugged her back.

"Oh, and Mel, in the age-old tradition of solidarity, we all took selfies too. And you, Ms. Debating Supergenius, have started a 'Brains over Beauty' movement that's gone viral and is rocking the national high school debate-team world."

He pulled out his phone and showed her the St. Petersburg Academy debate-team Facebook page. Every member had posted their own pics in some pretty awful bathing suit poses with captions:

"Beauty is fleeting but brains last forever."
"Clearly you can't rebuttal me out of this outfit."
"I maintain an affirmative argument that I am more than this
    picture."
"I can argue my way out of a paper bathing suit."
"I've got the power to use my words."

Mel cried and knew, without a doubt, she had found people who accepted and even valued all of her: her smart side, her argumentative side, her foodie side, her overweight side, and her music-loving side. She was more than those pictures and that, without question, was the real big fat truth.

3
Dadi's Chart

Lesley Jo Weaver

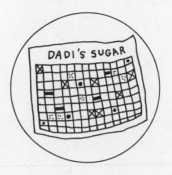

"Dadi's Chart" tells the story of Anjali, an eleven-year-old girl who decides to help her grandmother manage her type 2 diabetes. Type 2 diabetes is caused by a combination of lifestyle factors, like inactivity and eating an unhealthy diet, and genetic factors. Contrary to the common perception that hunger is the only nutrition-related problem in India, diseases related to overnutrition, like diabetes, are becoming big problems. More than 8 percent of the total population has diabetes, which is slightly higher than rates in the United States. Of all the chronic diseases, type 2 diabetes is one of the most complicated to manage because it requires precisely timed medicines, diet changes, exercise, and regular checkups at the doctor. Yet good illness management can help people avoid all kinds of complications associated with diabetes, such as kidney disease, vision loss, and heart problems. This story shows how family support can make all the difference in the management of a complicated illness.

Anjali got a big piece of paper from the stationer's store down the street from her house. She carefully drew vertical lines going down the entire page then changed the orientation of the ruler and drew horizontal lines. The result was a page full of little squares, except for a blank space at the top where a title would go. This was exactly what she wanted. Anjali then got some crayons and paints, which she used to make decorated labels for each column and row. Finally, she wrote at the top in big, bright letters, "Dadi's sugar."

This chart would help Anjali's grandmother, Dadi, remember to keep track of her diabetes. Dadi had been diagnosed a few months earlier with diabetes, or "sugar," as most people in New Delhi, India, called it. Like many women with diabetes in India, Dadi was having trouble taking care of herself.

Anjali often went with Dadi to the doctor, partially because in India, people believe it's a shameful thing for someone to be forced to go out alone, especially women. Besides, Anjali hoped to become a doctor one day, so she was always interested in seeing what doctors do. Whenever Dadi had to go to the doctor, she would wait for Anjali to come home from school and they would go together while her parents were still at work. Dadi's eyesight was not very good, so Anjali could help her step in and out of the auto rickshaw they took to the clinic and could help her haggle with the driver to get a fair price. While they were away, their maid, Sunita, always looked after the house and started dinner preparations. Most people in Delhi would not leave their maid alone in their home without supervision, but Sunita had been working for them since before Anjali was born, so they trusted her very much.

Anjali and Dadi had just come home from the doctor this afternoon. As Anjali put the finishing touches on the chart, she thought about how the doctor had checked Dadi's blood sugar using a finger-prick blood test, like always, and then gave her a stern lecture. "*Dekho*, Mrs. Mehra," he said in formal Hindi, peering at her over the top rim of his glasses as he reviewed her chart, "you have got to get your sugar under control. Right now you are only taking pills, but if you can't manage your blood sugar on these, we'll need to add insulin."

Dadi looked alarmed. "No, Doctor-sir, I could never take those injections!" she exclaimed.

"Most people feel that way at first, but they do become accustomed," he said. "Insulin is a very effective way to bring down blood sugar. I must tell you, Mrs. Mehra, that you are running serious risk of damaging your eyesight even further if you allow your sugar to continue being this high all the time. You could also have serious kidney or heart damage, and you're at high risk for skin infections. Type 2 diabetes is not to be taken lightly."

"What can I do?" she asked, a note of desperation in her voice.

"Well." The doctor paused, glancing Anjali's way, and sighed. "Diabetes is a complicated illness. In many ways, you have to become your own doctor when you have sugar. You must exercise, eat the kind of diet we discussed at your last appointment, and make sure to take your medicines. What's more, you need to do all of these things in an organized way, at specific times in the day, or else they might hurt you rather than help you. Actually," he said, pausing thoughtfully and glancing Anjali's way again, "we have had some success asking patients like you to elect a family member to help them manage all these things. One woman who was here last week asked her granddaughter to do it. We call these people health helpers. Anjali, do you think you could help your Dadi-ji in this way?"

Anjali loved her Dadi so much. Dadi had always lived with them, and she had helped raise Anjali from the time she was a baby. She and Anjali had special jokes only they knew—and even a secret hand sign they used to tell each other that Anjali's parents were crazy sometimes. She and Dadi would always laugh because Anjali's parents didn't get it. They had become especially close after Dada, her grandfather, passed away a few years ago.

"Yes, sir," Anjali said, sitting up straighter in her chair, "I think I could." After all, she already knew what Dadi was supposed to be doing to take care of herself. She always paid close attention when they went to the doctor.

"Good!" said the doctor.

Dadi smiled at her, patting her hand.

"You already know," the doctor continued, "about your Dadi-ji's diet, right? Do you still have the chart my dietician wrote for her?" Anjali nodded yes, remembering the detailed list of things that Dadi was supposed to eat every two hours.

"And you remember that she needs to take her medicine fifteen minutes before lunch and fifteen minutes before dinner?" Anjali nodded again. That was also written on the dietician's paper.

"Now, the next thing is that your Dadi-ji needs to lose some weight. She should go on a walk every day, and she should not eat more than one chai cup of rice a day. She should not take sugar in her milk or tea. No sweets, avoid potatoes, and—I'm sorry, Mrs. Mehra—no mangoes. They are so sweet that they could make your blood sugar go very high." Dadi loved mangoes, and mango season was coming. This would be hard for her, Anjali knew. But they had both heard this more than once; the doctor and the dietician had told them before.

"Finally, your Dadi-ji needs to start checking her blood sugar at home with a machine like this one," the doctor said, showing Anjali a thing that looked like a little, round mobile phone. "This is a new thing for her, but she needs to do it so we can see how high and how low her blood sugar is going every day. The company has given us some of these free blood sugar devices, so you can have this one to take home, but you still have to buy test strips and needles for it from the pharmacist. Many people do not like to do the finger stick themselves, so you can help your Dadi-ji with this. Make sure to test it once in the morning, before she eats anything, and once again two hours after breakfast. And write down what the machine says each time so that I can review it at her next appointment. OK?"

This was a lot of information to remember, but Anjali had heard most of it before. Only the blood testing was new to her, and she knew that their neighbor Ahmed, the local pharmacist, would help her learn how to do it.

"OK," Anjali said, nodding and thinking about her new responsibility.

Their talk with the doctor had taken place earlier in the afternoon, and now Anjali was finishing Dadi's chart. There was so much to keep track of, but she felt excited and very grown up when she thought of the idea that she could help keep Dadi from getting sick. Each row of the chart represented a day of the month, and the columns were labeled "first blood sugar," "second blood sugar," "walking time," "lunch medicine," "dinner medicine," "weight," and "good diet." Anjali would write down each of the day's two blood sugar readings in the first two columns, record the amount of time Dadi spent walking in the third one, make a check mark when she took her lunch and dinner medicines, and write down her weight in the "weight" column whenever they got it checked. Finally, she would place a gold star in the last column at the end of every day if Dadi stuck to her diabetic diet. Dadi would only get a gold star if she really did the diet, Anjali decided.

Anjali stuck the chart on the wall in the kitchen, and next to it she put up the paper from the dietician with Dadi's diet guidelines. Dadi was napping, but Anjali was so excited to show her the chart that she couldn't wait any longer. She went to Dadi's room and climbed into bed with her, hugging her around the neck and whispering, "Wake up, Dadi!"

Dadi's wrinkly eyes opened slowly, and she blinked, smiling. "My Gullu!" she said fondly, using the nickname she always called Anjali.

"Come on, Dadi! I have something to show you," said Anjali, jumping down from the bed and tugging Dadi's hand.

"See? It's your sugar chart!" she said, pulling Dadi into the kitchen. "Since I'm your health helper now, we need to keep track of all these things."

"Gullu, it's perfect!" said Dadi. "I love the colors."

"We'll write down everything until we see the doctor next month, then we'll take this chart with us so he can see it, all right?" said Anjali.

Dadi nodded, looking proudly at her Gullu.

"But first," Anjali continued, "we need to go see Ahmed to get the strips and needles for your blood sugar machine."

✦

Dadi tied up some money in the end of her pale pink sari and she and Anjali walked together out of their apartment and down the stairs, stepping over the dog who always laid in the entryway. When they got to Ahmed's shop, Anjali showed him the machine the doctor had given them. Ahmed produced two small boxes, one of test strips and one of needles, then showed Anjali how to put the test strip in the machine and how to put the needle in the finger-stick pen. When she pushed a button on the pen, it would automatically stick Dadi's finger, and she could even adjust how hard the prick was so that it would produce just the right amount of blood. Then she would touch the blood dot with the test strip, and it would suck the blood up for the test. Dadi said it didn't really hurt at all. The supplies were very expensive because they were imported, and it was only enough for fifty days' worth of twice-daily testing. Anjali packed up the new items in a little carrying case that had come with the blood sugar machine. On their way home, Anjali and Dadi speculated that maybe, if they did a good job with the monitoring this month, the doctor would tell her she could stop after a while.

The next morning, Anjali waited until she knew Dadi was finished with her morning *pooja* (prayer), then came in to check her blood sugar. Dadi didn't even flinch when Anjali pricked her with the needle. The machine said 154. Anjali wrote it on the chart. Then she and Dadi had a breakfast of *doodh daliya*, or milky porridge. When Dadi reached for the sugar bowl, Anjali said, "No, no, no, Dadi," wagging her finger in her best imitation of her mom. They both laughed at the impersonation, and Anjali got ready for school quickly.

At Anjali's school, most children went home for lunch. When Anjali came home at one o'clock that day, Dadi said she was not feeling very good. She had a headache. Anjali asked her if she had eaten the midmorning fruit snack she was supposed to have between breakfast and lunch, and Dadi confided that she had not. Did she check her blood sugar two hours after breakfast? No, again.

"Dadiiii!" Anjali protested. "There goes your gold star for the day. I'll have to get Sunita to help you while I'm away at school." Glancing at the chart, she remembered that Dadi needed her first medicine before lunch, so she gave it to her. A few minutes later, they had their lunch of *roti* and *sabji* (flatbread and vegetables) with *dal* (lentils). Anjali put Dadi's medicines in a basket on the dining table and placed it right in front of Dadi's seat so they would be there to remind her.

Later that evening, when Anjali came home from school, she talked with the maid, Sunita, about Dadi's eating schedule. Because she belonged to a low caste and was not educated, Sunita couldn't read, so Anjali explained what was written on the dietician's paper and asked her to make sure that Dadi ate a snack within two or three hours of finishing her breakfast and another between lunch and dinner. Then Anjali and Dadi went out for an evening walk at the park in their neighborhood. They saw lots of neighbors and chatted quite a lot. When the family sat down for dinner together, Anjali reminded Dadi to take her medicine and made a check in the box on the chart, but there was no gold star that day. "It's all right, Dadi," consoled Anjali. "It's just the first day."

Anjali went to bed that night thinking that being Dadi's health helper was an awful lot of work. But then again, she hoped, it might become easier once the routine got going.

And it did become easier as the days went by. Dadi started coming to Anjali's room directly after finishing her pooja for her morning blood test, and she started taking her medicines without being reminded. Sunita gave Dadi some fruit each morning at ten thirty sharp, and Dadi remembered that before she had the fruit, she needed to do her second blood test. The check marks and numbers started to fill up the chart. There were even some gold stars. Dadi didn't have any more headaches.

Finally, it was the end of the month and time to go back to the doctor. As usual, Anjali went along with Dadi, the chart rolled up under her arm. When she showed it to the doctor, he was very impressed.

"Wah, wah, Anjali," he said, approvingly. "This is really good. And look, your Dadi-ji's numbers have been going down a little bit," he said, pointing to the columns with the blood test readings. "That's really great."

When he checked Dadi's weight, he reported, pleased, that Dadi had lost a kilo (about two pounds) since her last visit. "Keep it up," he said, but he didn't tell Dadi that she could stop testing her blood sugar, as they had hoped he might.

Things proceeded in the same way for the next month, and Dadi's numbers continued to improve. When they returned to the doctor again, he said Dadi had lost another two kilos and that this weight loss would really help her to be healthier. Anjali beamed. He also ordered a blood test for Dadi, which would give him a better idea of her blood sugar changes in the previous two months. If it looked good, he said, Dadi could stop checking her blood sugar so often.

As it turned out, it did look good, so Dadi only had to check her blood sugar once a day from then on, and then just once a week. She started going to the doctor for checkups only once every three months. She and Anjali went on a walk together every day after school, and Anjali, too, felt more energetic with this routine. The whole family stopped eating desserts because they didn't want Dadi to feel bad, and even Anjali's papa began to lose a little weight. Everyone's doing better now that Dadi is doing better, thought Anjali. I'm so glad I could help her take care of herself.

4
Mai'suka, My Island

Kelley Alison Smith and Chandra Y. Osborn

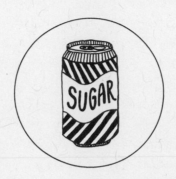

"Mai'suka, My Island" introduces the problems of overeating and poor nutrition, which contribute to obesity, type 2 diabetes, and strokes. These chronic conditions afflict people around the world and in particularly large numbers in American Samoa, an island territory of the United States located between Hawaii and New Zealand. In this story, Laea realizes that her friends' eating behaviors contribute to the problems that her mother and others in her community face by being overweight and having poor control of their blood sugar. Laea participates in a diabetes mentoring program so that she can educate and empower her peers to transform their behaviors and combat the increasing problem of obesity in her community.

FRIDAY

The Leone Lions were crushing the Kanana Fou Stallions at the football game at Tafuna Stadium. It was the third quarter and the score was 35 to 0. "Another blowout, you know?" Sefa and Tai and some other boys joked. They threw potato chips and cheese popcorn at each other, yelling, "Stallions suck!" The girls—Easter, 'Ata, and Laea among them—were starting to talk about how there must be something else to do.

"What else is there to do on a Friday night in American Samoa?" 'Ata asked. Pretty much everybody knew she was about to suggest that Sefa drive them all back out toward their village on the rugged west side of the island near Sliding Rock, where the sea crashes hard against the cliffs. They'd been there before, so they knew what would happen: Sefa would park his truck at that high spot on the road overlooking the ocean and 'Ata would drink one of those big Vailima beers too fast and then climb into the front seat of the truck with Sefa. Easter and Laea would sit on the matted green grass on the cliff, watching the moon and feeling the ground underneath rumble every time there was a big wave.

No one had any better ideas, as usual, so the choice was made to head to Sliding Rock. While walking out of the stadium, Sefa had to pull Tai off the brother of a Kanana Fou player who had heard him insulting the Stallions. Here, feuds over nonsense are a dime a dozen. Completely unfazed, Tai, 'Ata, Laea, and Easter made their way to Sefa's pickup, hopped in the back, and were off down the Ili'ili Road in the humid night, jostling over potholes.

Sefa had that "Airplanes" song cranked up loud, and everyone sang along. There are only two flights a week from Hawaii to Pago Pago, American Samoa's capital, most of the year. Three times a week in the summer. That's why a lot of people, especially the *palagi* (expatriate) crowd, call it the "Rock"—because it's literally an isolated rock in the middle of the South Pacific.

At Sliding Rock, Easter and Laea sat down on the grass, and 'Ata climbed out of the pickup bed and into the front seat, slamming the door behind her. Tai joined Easter and Laea, elbowing himself between them and draping his arms around their shoulders. Laea rolled her eyes and gave him his arm back.

"Come on, Laea, why you gotta be like that?" he protested. He sighed, collapsing his back onto the grass.

Easter took a can of Vienna sausages and a bag of cheese puffs out of her purse, pulled open the tab on the can of sausages, and threw the lid off the cliff. "Have one," she offered, reaching in herself.

"Umm, no thanks," Laea said, shaking her head in disgust. "I don't eat that stuff."

"Oh, but they taste so good."

"They're really bad for you," said Laea. "It's not even real meat. More like dog food—you know, meat by-products. Plus, they look like fat little fingers."

"Oh yeah, Laea?" said Tai, propping himself on his elbows. "Listen to you. Preach it, sister." She shoved his shoulder; his ample belly jiggled as he fell back to the ground in mock horror.

"Look, my mom has *mai'suka*," she said, referring to the "sugar disease," or diabetes.

"So she's not supposed to eat candy and cookies," Easter interrupted.

"It's not just candy," Laea said. "It's all this junk. All this artificial food loaded with fat and salt and chemicals to make it taste good. It's eating *pisupo* [tinned corned beef] and french fries and pineapple pie and bowls of ramen noodles and greasy barbecue. My mom knows she shouldn't eat it, but she does, and then sometimes she drinks so many sodas that she feels sleepy."

"Can't she just take medicine for that?" asked Easter. "I mean, I know a lot of Samoans with mai'suka, and they take pills to take care of it."

"Well, yeah, she can take medicine, but it's really expensive. And you know my dad's not working very much right now, since the tuna cannery cut back everybody's hours. But the point is that her doctor thinks she can keep her diabetes under control if she changes how she eats and starts getting some exercise. I'm trying to help her. Her doctor said if she doesn't start making changes, her diabetes could get so bad that she would have to go to the hospital every other day for the rest of her life so a dialysis machine can filter her blood. I just feel like, well, the way we Samoans eat now, it's slowly killing all of us."

"You want a quicker way to be killed?" Tai teased. "I can push you off this cliff right now. Death by Sliding Rock."

"Shut up, Tai," Laea said. "This is serious. Have you ever had your blood sugar checked?"

"Girl, I don't know what you're talking about. Pass me those cheese puffs," Tai said to Easter. "I'm seventeen. I'm supposed to eat this stuff!"

"Are you even hungry, Tai?" Laea snapped. "Or are you just eating crap because you're bored?"

He didn't answer.

"Well, I for one like these Vienna sausages," said Easter, helping herself to another one.

"You guys should come to Utulei Beach next Saturday morning," Laea said. "The health clinics on the island have all joined together and are going to check people's blood sugar and blood pressure for free. You know, test them to see if they're at risk for diabetes, talk about ways to eat better and what to do if you have diabetes. I volunteered to help. There's a meeting after school on Monday for people who want to be involved."

"Too bad I'm busy," said Tai.

A big wave crashed underneath the cliff and the truck door opened. 'Ata got out with her braid all messed up. "I'm ready to go home," Tai announced. "Preacher Laea here has been telling me and Easter about how bad our diets are, how we're all killing ourselves by eating cheese puffs. It's like she thinks we're drug addicts or something." He shook his head and glared at her. "You're just so much fun to hang with, Laea. So much fun. And you complain that you don't have a boyfriend."

"I've never complained . . ." Laea began but then stopped. "Whatever, Tai. Maybe some people just have to learn the hard way." She shrugged and climbed back into the bed of the truck.

At Laea's house her mom was watching TV, sitting on the sofa in a cotton muumuu printed with pink hibiscus flowers. Her ankles were swollen again, and she had her feet up. "How was the game, honey?" she asked, taking a sip of cola.

"Leone won again," said Laea, pausing for a moment. "Mom, why do you keep drinking that soda when you know how bad it is for your mai'suka and the doctor keeps telling you to stop? Let me get you some water instead."

"A few little sips won't hurt me." Her mom returned her attention to the TV.

MONDAY

Laea dragged a folding chair into the school lounge. A few other students were there.

Mrs. Sili, the English teacher, thanked everyone for coming. "I'm really glad to see you all here," she said. "Mai'suka is a big problem on this island. We all know people who have been affected by it. My sister and brother both have it. And it's going to affect our future if our community doesn't start making changes to the way we eat and live."

The students nodded shyly.

"Now, I know you're here because you want to volunteer next Saturday at Utulei, when we offer the free screenings for blood sugar and blood pressure," continued Mrs. Sili. "That's a good start, and I'm really glad that you all are going to help out with that. But what we're hoping to do is even more ambitious. We want to train volunteer community health workers—including young people like you—to help people manage their diabetes and take action to change their behaviors. I've agreed to coordinate the young people's volunteer program."

"But what if people don't want to change how they eat?" asked Laea. "I mean, my friends just get mad when I start talking about this stuff, even though some of them are really unhealthy."

"Not everyone wants to make changes," agreed Mrs. Sili. "The program we're establishing will recruit people with diabetes to participate. They have to want to be part of it. And if you decide that you want to become a community health worker, we'll train you to help people make better decisions about healthy eating, exercise, and getting medical care when they need it."

"Why would somebody listen to me?" asked a boy named Opu. "Why wouldn't they just take their doctor's advice?"

"Well, that's a good question," said Mrs. Sili with a smile. "Let me ask you something: have your parents or your doctor ever given you advice you didn't take?"

Opu laughed and nodded.

"I won't ask you what that advice was," she said, and everyone chuckled. "Listen, people say they want to make changes to how they live. But it's one thing to say it and it's another thing to do it. And sometimes people get embarrassed. They don't want their doctor to think they're stupid because they eat too much at a wedding or forget to take a pill sometimes. So this program will help people with diabetes to set goals that are achievable. And the community health workers will visit these people every couple of weeks to give them support and encouragement. It won't be a substitute for getting medical care when they need it."

"But I couldn't tell someone older, especially a man, how to take care of himself," a girl named Fasa pointed out. "I mean, that is just not *fa'a Samoa* [the Samoan way]. Older people would think I was being rude."

"The idea is that we would match you up with people your own age and your own sex," said Mrs. Sili. "If you decide you want to participate, we'll help teach you how to answer some of those questions. Now," she continued, "I already told you that my brother and sister have diabetes. Let me tell you about my father. He is a *matai* [chief] in our village who likes to tell stories. At sixty-two years old, he boasts that he can still spear bigger fish more quickly than most men one-third his age. I don't know if that's true, but he talks about what life on the island was like when he was younger. 'We walked to school every day,' he says. 'None of this driving these big trucks! No one had cars! If we were hungry, we stopped to pick bananas and papayas from the trees. And we had drinks from *niu* [young coconuts] when we were thirsty.'"

"You know," Mrs. Sili said, leaning forward in her folding chair, "my father tells this story over and over again when he sees his descendants mindlessly stuffing themselves full of chips and soda in front of the television or complaining that they don't have flashier cars. And he says that we Samoans used to be warriors, muscular and strong." She shook her head. "I wonder about it myself. I look at the matais and elders I know, and while some of them are big, most of them are slender, like my father. I look around at choir practice in church sometimes and wonder how potato chips and pickup trucks have made us obese and so prone to mai'suka in just a couple of generations. I don't want it to happen to me, and I don't want it to keep happening to the people on my island."

Laea thought it was odd to hear a teacher speak like this. Usually teachers were yelling at the class to pay attention and for the boys to quit drawing outlines of breasts with their hands. Laea liked Mrs. Sili, liked that she wasn't afraid to tell them about her own family.

After the meeting, Laea helped put the folding chairs away. "Thank you for coming, Laea," Mrs. Sili said. "It seems like you really care about this issue."

"Yeah," Laea admitted. "My mom has mai'suka."

"Does she take good care of herself?" Mrs. Sili asked kindly.

"Not really." Laea shook her head.

"Do you want to tell me about it?"

"Well, I guess. You're not going to tell my mom I told you this, right?" Laea asked.

"Of course not," Mrs. Sili reassured her.

Laea tried to find the words that would convey her concern without being disrespectful. "My mom went to Leone High too. And people still talk about how she was such a great volleyball player, back when she wasn't big and unhealthy like she is now. Last summer I played on the church volleyball team and everybody was like, 'That was good, Laea, but, oh! You should have seen your mother once upon a time.'"

Mrs. Sili nodded for her to continue.

"We had a big family reunion last summer too, and people flew in from Western Samoa and from Hawaii and California and even Alaska—I mean, you know how these reunions are, it's like everybody who arrives on the island is related to you."

Mrs. Sili smiled.

"Anyway, there were some fierce volleyball games at the fields at Lions Park. So Auntie Ipo finally talked my mom into joining one, and Mom took a big Styrofoam container of barbecue, chop suey, and pie off her lap and she sighed and went over to join the game. But only five minutes later she was totally out of breath. She bent over with her hands on her knees, and then she excused herself. Everyone was polite about it, but I saw Uncle Teʻo and Cousin Eni roll their eyes and shake their heads. People said, 'It's OK, it's OK, Auntie,' trying to make her feel better. Finally my cousin asked me to come over and help cool Mom off by waving a fan. And I got over and started fanning her and she was drinking a soda."

"That sounds really hard," said Mrs. Sili.

"It's not that I'm embarrassed by her, exactly." Laea thought for a moment. "I mean, I respect her. She's my mom. It's more that I think she's smart, right? But then she makes really bad choices about this stuff."

"I think she's lucky to have a daughter who cares this much about her health." Mrs. Sili escorted Laea out of the lounge. "Thanks so much for coming. I'm glad to have you be part of this program, Laea."

"Thank you, too, for listening," said Laea. "It just never seems like the right time to talk to her about it, and I'm afraid we're running out of time."

"Then we've got a lot of work to do," said Mrs. Sili. "I'll see you at the health screenings at Utulei, and we'll get started."

5

Thiago and the Beach

Brian Ackerman

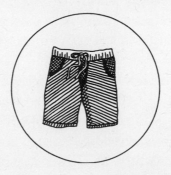

"Thiago and the Beach" reveals a young man's journey as he learns to accept who he is, both inside and out. For years, Thiago struggled with his weight and with fitting in. His negative image of his body often prevents him from living a normal life and participating in events like going to the beach. His image of what a young gay guy should look like—fit and thin— make it difficult for him to accept himself and his overweight body. Thiago's friendship with Mariana enables him to face his fears—that people are judging him or not accepting him for not having an idealized body—and his persistent anxiety over feeling like an outcast. This story introduces an uncommonly discussed challenge of growing up gay, as body image is a sig- nificant part of many gay adolescents' sense of self-worth as they begin to seek acceptance from the gay community. It is Thiago's social relationships that give him strength to be himself and to accept who he is amid discrimi- nation and fear of nonacceptance by society.

It's never going to get any better, is it? Thiago thought. He was in the store dressing room trying on a new pair of board shorts as he looked himself up and down in the mirror. He was thinking about his weight as he surveyed his whole body.

Though he was five feet ten inches tall, he weighed almost 230 pounds. He cringed at the sight of his waistline—his belly and sides bulging over the top of the shorts. Even looking at his hands, his fingers seemed like they were swollen. His face was bloated and covered with small acne breakouts—red and white bumps peeking out from under the skin. He did not feel *lindo* (cute) or *gatinho* (hot) or any of those things that everyone seemed to consider important for a young gay guy.

Then he thought about Sunday, just a few days away. His friend Mariana, who had recently come out as a lesbian, invited him to come to the gay beach with her in Ipanema. Being from the North Zone of Rio de Janeiro, Mariana and Thiago did not frequent the South Zone beaches, except on holidays and those weekends they were able to make the trek on the trains and buses they needed to get there. Thiago loved the beach, probably more than anywhere else, but as he got older, he went less and less, even though as a teenager his mom was letting him go out more on his own.

So when Mariana, who had known him since primary school, invited him, she knew it would be a struggle. "Come on!" she said over instant messenger, trying to convince him to go. "It will be fun! And there are so many *gatos* [hot guys] there that you have to meet!"

Mariana's excitement over the gay beach was understandable. Throughout the country, at least one person is killed every day for being gay, lesbian, bisexual, or transgender. Even though Rio is widely recognized for being a gay-friendly city, violence is not a thing of the past. Few places in the whole country are as gay friendly as the one stretch of sand on Ipanema beach where the multicolored gay pride flag waves in the ocean wind.

For Cariocas, people from the city of Rio de Janeiro, the beach is like a backyard; it is the place where everyone in the city—rich, poor, gay, straight, black, white, and mulatto—comes together and shares a single space without any of the concrete walls and barbed-wire barriers that demarcate boundaries between people in the rest of the city.

Interestingly enough, even in the absence of these boundaries, the Cariocas have designed a way to separate the long stretches of sand into specific areas—the subtle presence of lifeguard posts and a few flags dotted along brings a unique culture to each location. There are different areas for surfers, for families from the North Zone, for soccer players, for older people from the South Zone, and most important to Thiago, for gay people.

The gay beach in Ipanema is one of the few gay-friendly spaces in the city that costs nothing to enter, that has no dress code, and that makes a clear statement to the rest of Rio de Janeiro that heterosexuality is not the only type of sexuality in Brazilian society. It is, in certain ways, an important space to feel a part of when growing up gay in Rio. Thiago had passed by it while walking on the boardwalk, but he had never spent the day there. When he went to the beach, it was with his family, when he was little. He was *gordinho* (little fat guy) then too, but that was never cause for self-consciousness within his family.

As a teenager, the gay beach in Ipanema can also feel very exclusive—only certain body types seem to be welcome. It is inhabited by some of the most toned and fit bodies one can imagine, with seemingly perfect muscles, great tans, and fancy hairdos. It's a place where anyone can feel excluded if they let the scenery determine their fate.

This was why Thiago was less than enthusiastic about Mariana's invitation. On Sundays the beaches are packed. It was summer too, which meant there would be even more people. But he did say yes to her—partly because he knew it would make her happy and partly because he actually did want to go.

As he kept looking at himself in the mirror in the dressing room, he felt a swell of anxiety as he realized the terrifying possibility that he would be the butt of someone's joke simply because of his weight. As he got older, Thiago noticed that his feelings of anxiety increasingly stopped him from doing things he wanted to do.

What if a group of them starts to make fun of me? he thought. He started to take off the board shorts and began to think he would have to cancel on Mariana. It was too much pressure. He was not one of those guys and never would be. Thiago thought that even on a beach, where just about everyone in Rio can find a place that feels like home, he would be rejected by the very community he sought support from most of all—all because of how he looked. He thought about the images of the few gay people he had seen on TV and in movies—they all seemed to be thin and have perfect smiles. While he had come out of the closet to some members of his family and close friends, he felt like his body was keeping him from really becoming part of the gay community.

Mariana popped up next to the dressing room. "So! How does it look? Are you going to look hot on Sunday?" she asked him, yelling over the door.

Thiago was silent.

"Oh, don't tell me you are thinking of not going. We came all the way to the mall to get new bathing suits so we will look good at the beach," she said.

Thiago, already changed out of the board shorts, opened the dressing room door with a melancholy look on his face. "I just don't think . . . um . . . I think I have something to do with my mom on Sunday so I can't go. I'm sorry. I forgot to tell you."

"Oh yeah? What do you have to do?" asked Mariana, suspicious of Thiago's sudden new priority.

"I have to . . . help her make beans. You know, it's a whole process and she needs some extra help," Thiago replied, increasingly confident in the story he was concocting on the spot.

"Oh right, you can't go to the beach on Sunday because you have to stay at home and help your mother make beans," said Mariana, sarcastically. "Is that really the best you could come up with? Let me translate that story for you: 'My name is Thiago. I didn't like how I looked in the board shorts I just tried on, so now instead of going to the beach and having fun, I will sit at home and tell my friends I am making beans with my mom.'"

Thiago's face quickly broke into a grin. Mariana's honesty was his favorite thing about her. She never let him back down from challenges, and she pushed him to push himself. They were a good pair.

"Well, you try being the fat gay guy around all those perfect people!" he responded defiantly.

"Oh, that's what this is about," said Mariana. "So what? You are a gordinho. I know it can be tough there—everyone is just trying to show off how they look. But it's more than that—it's a place where you can feel safe to be who you are."

"It's a place where you feel safe if you look perfect. It's not a place that I feel safe. The beach is scary for me, Mariana. I love the beach, but I don't like that I feel so ugly."

"Listen to yourself! You love the beach. What does that mean? You should go to places you love. If the beach is one of them, then go enjoy it. Everyone there is too obsessed with themselves to be concerned about how you look."

"But I want them to like me," Thiago responded, admitting what his fear was really about. "I want to be one of those guys who goes to the beach who everyone thinks is beautiful. I know you're right, most people there are more focused on themselves than on everyone around them, but I can't help feeling self conscious."

With a small smile, Mariana gently grabbed Thiago's arm and said, "Do you like you? Do you think you're beautiful?"

"No. I mean, well, I wish I was, but I'm not," he said.

"Well then, we've had a breakthrough! You are not scared of the beach, you are scared of yourself!" exclaimed Mariana. "You want those guys to look at you and think you're beautiful? Then make yourself something you think is beautiful. Beautiful is a lifestyle. Those thin guys and the ones with the muscles work out every day because they think that's what health and beauty is. If you think that's what it is, you can get your body in shape too. But don't sit around and avoid the beach, the place you love, because you are scared of your potential to be as beautiful as anyone there. No one can take that potential away from you, and no one can take the beach from you. You have just as much a right to be there as anyone else, no matter what you look like in a bathing suit."

Thiago was silent as he looked down at the board shorts he had just tried on and was now gripping tightly in his hands. He felt that cool sensation in the pit of his stomach and beads of sweat emerging on his forehead.

"So, do you still have to cook beans on Sunday?" said Mariana.

"It's not that easy," said Thiago, conscious of how anxious the thought of going to the beach made him.

"What's not that easy?"

"You talk about how I can be as beautiful as I want, and that I belong there just as much as anyone else. But you're beautiful; girls and guys love you. You already had a boyfriend and a girlfriend. You don't understand. I'm fat. I'm ugly. I can't just make that feeling go away."

"Thiago, if you can't make that feeling go away, then who can? I'm not saying it will go away tomorrow, or even by Sunday when we go to the beach, but if you want to be 'that beautiful guy on the beach' then you have to decide what 'beautiful Thiago' looks like and be that. But staying at home and making beans probably won't get you there."

"Uh-huh," Thiago murmured.

"So board shorts, yes or no?" said Mariana.

"Yessss, I'm getting them," Thiago whined, admitting he was convinced by Mariana's arguments.

"*Puxa! Que legal!* [Yay! Very cool!]," exclaimed Mariana. "It's going to be great."

Over the next few days, Thiago repeatedly tried on the board shorts in his room. Examining himself in the mirror each time, he tried to envision what "beautiful Thiago" looked like. He imagined what he would look like if he were skinnier, muscular even. He thought about what he would have to do to be that way. To him, it just seemed like all those beautiful people were just naturally like that—that their image was effortless. He felt overwhelmed and kept thinking that he would have to cancel on Mariana again.

He sent her a text message on Sunday morning: "Hey Mari! Feeling a little sick, don't think I can go 2day."

He waited for her to respond but heard nothing. He thought about sending the message again. Then he thought she might be upset with him.

After a few minutes there was a knock at the door. Thiago's mom called him to say it was Mariana. Thiago walked to the door in his pajamas to greet Mariana, who was all ready with her sunscreen and a *kanga* (beach towel).

"Where are your board shorts?!"

"I just sent you a—"

"Yeah, I got it," interrupted Mariana. "I thought you might cancel on me, so I decided to come and get you. I'm going to the beach today. Are you coming?" she said.

Thiago thought for a moment while he looked down at the floor.

"Ugh. Fine," he said. "But if this doesn't go well I am going to blame you!"

"Great, blame whoever you want, but we have a bus to catch!"

Thiago and Mariana kissed Thiago's mom good-bye and headed for the bus stop. The journey from their neighborhood to Ipanema beach took about an hour, even on Sunday when traffic was light. The fifteen-minute bus ride took them to the metro stop in Pavuna, a suburb of Rio de Janeiro, where they got on a train that would take them all the way to Ipanema.

As the train inched closer to Zona Sul, the South Zone, Thiago became a bit more anxious. He noticed his reflection in the window across from him and was reminded of how ugly he felt. By the time the two reached Ipanema, he didn't want to get off the train.

"All right, we made it!" said Mariana, as she grabbed her things to walk toward the door of the train car.

Thiago summoned the courage to give a half smile, despite his nerves, and reluctantly followed.

When they arrived on the beach, Thiago was excited to see the unique square design of the black-and-white marble mosaic on the Ipanema *calçadão* (boardwalk). He loved this place. Mariana tugged at his arm and pointed at the beach.

"See! There it is," she said, directing Thiago's eyes toward the gay pride flag waving in the wind above the canopy of umbrellas shading beachgoers from the sun.

They kicked off their sandals and felt the scorching heat of the sand on their feet.

"Ow!" Mariana yelled.

"Caramba!" Thiago responded, as they walked briskly toward the masses of people camped on the sand.

Mariana led the way, toting her kanga in her beach bag and smiling back at Thiago. Sidestepping the arms, legs, and heads sticking out into their makeshift path, they walked until they were directly under the flag, next to the stand that rented chairs and umbrellas.

Thiago's heart was racing. All he could think about was the question Mariana would ask him once they sat down: When was he going to take off his shirt? He looked around, anxiously waiting for people making fun of him, this heavy adolescent, as he ungracefully trudged through the sand looking for a spot that would fit his frame.

"How about here?" Mariana called out when she had come to an open clearing in the sand.

Out of breath and sweating profusely, Thiago nodded his head and said, "Uh-huh."

They spread out their kangas on the sand and Mariana shimmied off her shorts and shirt, revealing a lime-green and black bikini underneath. Thiago stood there, frozen.

"Did you put on sunscreen already?" asked Mariana.

"No, I mean, not really, I don't think so," Thiago responded. He was nervous, that much was clear. He had thought about this moment a million times.

"You don't think so? Well, let me put some on your back then so you don't turn into a *camarão*!" (Camarão, which means "big shrimp," is a nickname friends call one another when they get a bad sunburn.) Mariana reached for her sunscreen bottle.

Thiago's stomach was in knots, but he started to peel off his shirt, which at that point was sticking to his skin from perspiration.

At that moment, a curious thing happened. Thiago realized that no one was making fun of him. Those around them hadn't even stopped their conversations. He had a revelation: almost all of the fear he had about not being able to fit in was in his head—which meant it was something he could control and change by understanding his fears better. As Mariana started to put sunscreen on his back, he looked around, noticing that there were bodies of all types at the beach, even people who were bigger, like him. He realized that while his weight made him different, it didn't make him any less of a person or any less of a gay person.

When they both laid down on their kangas, Thiago clued Mariana into what he was thinking. "This isn't what I was expecting," he said.

"Well, what did you have in mind? Whatever it was it seemed pretty intimidating," Mariana responded.

"I just thought I would feel so ugly here, like I didn't belong, because of my weight. But it's not like that. Everyone is just kind of enjoying the beach," he said.

"Of course they are! That's why people come. Not to care about how everyone else looks. You are at the best beach in Brazil, and I get to be here with my best friend. I'm so glad you came," said Mariana, smiling.

Thiago kept thinking about what Mariana had said a few days earlier, about him having to think about what it meant to him to be beautiful. He realized he needed to identify what he wanted to change about himself. He had always wanted to be a *magrinho* (skinny guy), but being skinny or fat wasn't really the issue. More important, he realized he had grown to consider his weight and his body to be the most important measurement of his value as an individual.

Thiago had been conditioned for so long—through the media, through name-calling, through his own thoughts—to think that he was somehow less worthy of being a part of the gay community. He hadn't even thought about working out because he thought only the beautiful people did that. He realized he wasn't just scared of going to the beach but of going to the gym, going on runs, and taking part in tons of activities he thought were reserved for the "beautiful guys."

Because he did not look like the ideal image of a gay teenager—thin and fit—he had accepted gordinho as his identity, instead of building a sense of self that was based on his talents and accomplishments. The childhood memories of his peers ignoring him because of his weight had stuck with him. But that day at the beach with Mariana, he saw there was a place for him in the gay community regardless of his body size. He realized that the past was past. If he wanted to change the future of his body, he could, but his body itself did not define his value as a person.

The Gay-Straight Alliance Network
Kathy Wollner

The Gay-Straight Alliance Network (GSA Network) is "a national youth leadership organization that connects school-based Gay-Straight Alliances (GSAs) to each other and community resources through peer support, leadership development, and training."[*] The network supports young people in the United States to start, strengthen, and maintain GSAs at their schools.

GSAs provide an important safe space for lesbian, gay, bisexual, transgender, queer, or questioning (LGBTQ) young people during the coming-out process, which takes place when, for example, a boy decides to tell a family member or friend that he is gay. GSAs bring LGBTQ students and their allies together, creating school communities where LGBTQ students are safer and school environments are more accepting. GSAs do this by supporting each other and learning about homophobia (discrimination based on sexual orientation), transphobia (discrimination based on gender identity), and other oppressions. After educating themselves, students share information about these issues with their classmates. An extremely important part of GSAs' work is fighting discrimination, harassment, and violence in schools.

We know from research that young people who are harassed because of their sexual orientation (being gay, lesbian, bisexual, queer, or questioning) have weaker connections to school and less support from teachers and other adults. They miss school more often and are more likely to be victims of violence. On the other hand, research from California shows that students with GSAs at their school feel safer and more supported.

The GSA Network, originally only in California, now works

---

[*] "Mission," Gay-Straight Alliance Network, 2009, accessed May 19, 2013, http://www.gsanetwork.org/about-us.

throughout the United States. The California organization has supported other states in starting their own networks, and there are now thirty-seven state networks throughout the country. The GSA Network has developed excellent resources to help students start GSAs, improve their schools' clubs, gain more members and allies, raise funds, speak publicly, and deal with apathy or opposition.

Do you feel inspired to start a GSA at your school? Here are "10 Steps for Starting a GSA," adapted from the GSA Network website:

1. Follow guidelines: start a GSA just like you would start another student group. Look in your student handbook for the rules.

2. Find a faculty advisor: find a teacher or staff member whom you think would be supportive or has already shown themselves to be an ally.

3. Tell the administration of your plans: tell administrators what you are doing right away. It can be very helpful to have an administrator on your side. If an administrator is resistant to the GSA, let them know that forming a GSA club is protected under the federal Equal Access Act.*

4. Tell guidance counselors and social workers about the group: they may know students who would be interested in attending the group.

5. Pick a meeting place: you may want to find a meeting place that is off the beaten path at school.

6. Advertise: figure out the best way to advertise at your school. It may be a combination of school bulletin announcements, flyers, and word of mouth. Also get food—people always come to meetings when there's food! If your flyers are drawn on or torn down, do not be discouraged. Keep putting them back up. Eventually, whoever is tearing them down will give up.

7. Hold your meeting: you may want to start out with a discussion

---

* The Equal Access Act, passed in 1984, is a federal law that compels secondary schools that receive federal funding to provide equal access to extracurricular clubs. This law has been essential in defending the right of students to form GSAs in court.

about why people feel having this group is important. You can also brainstorm things your club would like to do during the school year.

8. Establish ground rules: many groups have ground rules in order to ensure that group discussions are safe, confidential, and respectful. Many groups have a ground rule that no assumptions are made or labels are used about a group member's sexual orientation or gender identity. This can help make allies feel comfortable attending the club.

9. Plan for the future: develop an action plan. Brainstorm activities. Set goals for what you want to work toward. Contact Gay-Straight Alliance Network in order to get connected to all of the other GSAs, get supported, and learn about what else is going on in the community.

10. Register your GSA: now that you've started it up, register your GSA with the GSA network in your state.

DISCUSSION QUESTIONS

- Do you have a GSA at your school? If so, how does it affect students and your school environment?

- If you don't have a GSA at your school, consider what might be different about how school usually runs if you were to have one.

- Name some possible barriers to creating a GSA in your school.

- How do GSAs support LGBTQ students? If you identify as LGBTQ, how would having an organization like this at school make you feel? If you don't, imagine yourself in another person's shoes: if you did identify in that way, how would you feel?

- What does it mean to be an ally?

- Identify two ways that a GSA can improve a school's environment for not only LGBTQ students but all students.

This section's information has been adapted from the GSA Network's website. To learn more about the GSA Network, to access its resources, and to see how you can get involved, visit www.gsanetwork.org.

Section II

Gender & Sexuality

S exuality is a fundamental part of living a healthy life. The World Health Organization defines *sexual health* as "a state of physical, emotional, mental and social well-being in relation to sexuality. . . . Sexual health requires a positive and respectful approach to sexuality and sexual relationships."[*] Many issues encompass sexual health, such as positive body image, sexual orientation, gender, and reproduction. We begin to grapple with sexual health issues early in life and experience them throughout our lives.

As humans, the body's normal process is to go through puberty during adolescence, but individuals begin puberty at different times. Girls usually go through puberty earlier than boys do, and girls and boys experience different changes to their bodies. While girls experience the development of breasts and the beginning of their menstrual cycle, boys experience testicular growth and changes in their voice. Puberty involves growth in height and new hair growth for both girls and boys, and it often includes emotional shifts and challenges as hormones change in the body. For many young people, this is also when a desire for romantic relationships with others begins or grows and when decisions about if and when to have sex are first made. Unfortunately, sex education is sometimes lacking in schools, and teenagers often make their decisions without knowledge of how to prevent pregnancy and sexually transmitted infections (STIs) or without access to birth control and condoms to act on the knowledge they do have. Everyone experiences puberty and adolescence in her or his own way.

Gender and sexuality can shape how people grow to understand who they are in relation to their family, school, social groups, and world. Some people find at an early age that the social roles to which they were born present unforeseen challenges. This is an important challenge and

* World Health Organization, "Defining Sexual Health," report of a technical consultation on sexual health, January 28–31, 2002, Geneva, Switzerland, http://www.who.int/reproductivehealth/publications/sexual_health/defining_sexual_health.pdf.

necessitates defining the difference between sex and gender. One's sexual organs—uterus, ovaries, and vagina for females, penis and testicles for males—define a person's sex. In this way, *sex* is biological. In contrast, *gender* is social. This means that it is not our sex that defines how we interact with the world; it is our gender. That's why we become who we are through our interaction with the world around us as well as through our predetermined biology.

Different cultures hold different measures of what it means to become a man or woman. For example, adolescents of Jewish descent present at bar mitzvahs (for boys at the age of thirteen) and bat mitzvahs (for girls at the age of twelve or thirteen). After these religious ceremonies, young people take on new roles and esteem within the Jewish community. Other cultures hold different types of coming-of-age ceremonies for adolescents. We bring up the complicated issue of female circumcision in this book, an initiation ceremony that occurs in some societies (the Maasai are one example), in order to illustrate how such ceremonies may differ across cultures. The practice of female circumcision involves the cutting of a female's external genitalia, as described in "Nditai's Initiation." While some people consider these ceremonies to be fundamental cultural traditions, others believe they are abusive and that girls should be protected from undergoing them under international human rights law. This is a very difficult and complicated topic.

Social norms—what society generally expects from people—determine what is dominant or most common in a culture. But these things can change over time. For example, same-sex relationships, such as between two men or two women, once lacked acceptance in the United States. Slowly such relationships are becoming recognized as acceptable, common, and healthy relationships. Yet people who are gay, lesbian, and bisexual are still judged or treated poorly by many people who discriminate against them based on their sexual orientation. Another example is that social norms tell us that a person's gender should be based on his or her sexual organs. However, some people who are born female feel like boys or men, and some people who are born males feel like girls or women. Such people are transgender. We discuss some of these feelings in "Chris Not Christina."

Women face unique challenges because the ability to bear children plays a special role in women's lives. While men play a role in reproduction, they will never experience childbirth for themselves or risk becoming pregnant when they are not yet ready to parent. In poor societies, where they may not be able to obtain health care, many women die during childbirth because they do not have access to a hospital or their health-care providers do not have the training or tools to address a complicated birth. This rarely happens in wealthy countries such as the United States, where there is better infrastructure and access to hospitals; however, some women in poor communities still face barriers to health care during their pregnancy, leading to lower rates of prenatal care in poor communities. Also, women face unique challenges as their bodies change significantly during pregnancy and after childbirth and they take on important new jobs, such as breastfeeding.

This section describes the ways in which gender and sexuality can shape how people see the world and their health. We begin this section with "Slow Motion," a story that illustrates the challenges associated with puberty. Then "Nditai's Initiation" brings to light the cultural and social issues surrounding female circumcision in Tanzania. The story "Chris Not Christina" introduces a young person who has never quite felt right living in a female body. In "Ariana's Decision," a young woman struggles with having sex for the first time and discovering she is pregnant. Finally, "My Body, My Self" describes a teenager who has a premature baby and must learn how to breastfeed him to enrich his health and their bond.

As you read through this section, think about the following questions:

- What changes do girls and boys experience during puberty?
- Do you think it would be difficult to live life as a different gender? What challenges might you face that are similar to or different from those that you face today?
- How do you think a woman feels when she finds out she is pregnant when that wasn't her plan? What challenges do young people face when having children in their teens? Also, what are the benefits of breastfeeding a baby?

6

Slow Motion

Patrick Klacza

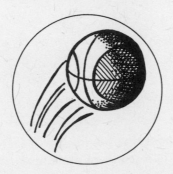

"Slow Motion" introduces Matt, a fourteen-year-old young man who is frustrated that he hasn't yet matured like his peers. While it seems everyone else has grown and sprouted new patches of hair, Matt still feels like a boy. Matt also struggles to discover what he wants for himself, in spite of pressure from his dad to play and succeed at basketball. This story explores the near-universal experience of puberty and shows how the reality of puberty differs for each person. While some young people go through puberty without too much thought, it can cause a great deal of stress for those who feel they are being left behind. By the story's end, Matt has learned an important lesson: he must live his own life, not the one his dad has laid out for him.

Late into the fourth quarter, Matt pressed the opposing guard, put a hand in his face, and shuffled with him past half court. The score was tied. He could feel the gym shake as fans stomped their feet on the old wooden bleachers. It was sticky hot and sweat ran down his face.

"Play D, guys," he said. "No cheap fouls."

This was no scrimmage game, no shirts versus skins. This was it: the eighth-grade semifinals, winner to play Eisenhower in the championship. The Spartans hadn't been to the finals in a decade, hadn't won it all in two. Coach Baker wanted so badly to win that he had started giving long, impassioned speeches in the locker room. When Matt shadowed the other guard—last name Riley—down the sideline, Baker was pacing like a man possessed, his face as red as Matt's jersey.

From the top row of the bleachers, Matt's dad watched the game through a video camera. He followed his son's every move. Matt rolled around a pick, trailed Riley to the corner, stopped, and ran back to the top of the key. On the camera's four-inch screen, a tiny version of Matt swiped at the ball, somehow got a finger on it, and stole it away.

Matt dribbled past Riley, and with another step, he was on a fast break. Mere seconds were left on the game clock. He could win it with a lay-up. No problem, he thought. Easiest shot in basketball. He jumped, aimed for the sweet spot on the backboard, and shot. His momentum carried him past the basket. He didn't see the ball go in, but judging from the roar, he knew it had.

Matt's dad had the camera all set up. He pressed play, and last night's game flickered onto the TV screen. "Pay attention," he said. "Here. See how you stumble? You've got to be quick."

"I hit the game winner."

"Season's not over. Learn from your mistakes, and you won't make them in the championship."

"I've got homework."

"This is your homework."

Matt watched himself sink shot after shot. In the third quarter, he hit a jumper from ten feet out to put the Spartans in the lead. His dad paused the video. Matt stood frozen post-follow-through, his arm in the air, his wrist loose.

Matt hated watching himself on the big screen. He was already self-conscious of how short he was, and seeing video proof of his scrawny body and fragile twig legs made him feel worse.

"You've got to box out," Dad said.

"I'm too short to get rebounds."

"Then get growing."

Matt wanted so badly to grow. His teammates had already hit puberty. They'd sprouted armpit air, leg hair, and, presumably, pubic hair. They'd grown Adam's apples, suffered growing pains in their shins, begun treating their oily, pimply skin. But not Matt. As he watched himself score the winning basket, he thought only about the shame of being hairless. He was the only boy on a team of young men.

On the day of the championship, Matt put on his uniform in a bathroom stall. The other guys were already dressed and waiting for Coach Baker. Matt slipped his jersey over his head and lifted his arms for inspection. No surprise, no hair. He'd been inspecting his pits every day for months, longing for the hair to grow.

He took off his jersey, found the undershirt he had stuffed into his duffel bag that morning, and put it on. He'd never worn sleeves beneath his jersey before. He felt constricted, but constriction was better than humiliation.

Throughout the game, Matt worried that his sleeves were getting in the way. He'd shoot, and they'd get stuck on his biceps, messing with his release. He couldn't buy a bucket, and in the end, Eisenhower pulverized the Spartans, 55–23. Nobody was on. Colby shot twenty, maybe thirty air balls. Jack kept dribbling out of bounds. Coach Baker looked like he'd hemorrhage out and collapse on the floor. But Matt played the worst, or at least that's how it felt. When he got home, he bypassed his dad, who had already set up the video camera, and went straight for the shower.

While scrubbing his shameful, stunted body, Matt cried. The whistling of the showerhead obscured the sound, and soapy water carried his tears down the drain. Excepting his bedroom—and even that was a dangerous place to cry, for fear of his dad discovering him—the shower was the only place he could let out how he was feeling. When he got it out of his system, he checked himself in the mirror, made sure his eyes were clear, and went downstairs to face his dad.

"Dad," he said, "I'm sick of this. When am I going to grow? When will I have some hair?"

"Remember when we talked about seeing a doctor?"

"Yes."

"I've still got his number."

"Well, let's go."

"All right. I'll call first thing in the morning."

In hopes of kick-starting his dormant pituitary gland, Matt and his dad had talked about starting Matt on a hormone regimen. Matt's dad had done some preliminary research on the Internet, and he thought Matt was a good candidate. A week after basketball season ended, Matt found himself in the waiting room at the doctor's office, bored and diagnosing strangers. That kid's cough doesn't sound real; he's faking sick to skip school.

When the nurse called his name, he trailed his dad into a tiny examination room. Like all the exam rooms that had come before, this one was white, orderly, and sterile. There was nothing to do in it but look at some boring posters and dream of licking the tongue depressors. After what seemed like hours spent waiting, someone knocked at the door and came in, manila folder in hand.

"My name's Dr. Brenner," said the man, and he sat at the computer and got right to typing. "What brings you in, Matt?"

"He's not growing, doc," said Matt's dad.

"I see." Dr. Brenner consulted his chart. "It says here he wants hormones."

"Wants? More like needs."

"Matt, is this what you want?"

Matt shifted his weight. The paper on the examining table crinkled. "I think so."

"Then I'll need to do a quick checkup. Mr. Stevens, it's my practice to do checkups with young men on their own, without their parents. I'll have my nurse come get you when we're finished."

When Matt's dad left the room, Dr. Brenner closed the door behind him. "What's this all about, Matt? You really want to take hormones?" he asked.

"I'm not growing. I'm short. I've got no hair."

"It's common for young men to just be starting puberty at your age. Have you noticed any changes?"

"I don't think so."

Dr. Brenner put on a pair of latex gloves.

"One thing I can do is examine your testicles. If they seem like they're growing, that's a good sign."

Matt groaned. No one likes a testicular exam.

"I know, I know," said Dr. Brenner. "It'll be quick. I swear."

Matt dropped his pants. He felt Dr. Brenner's cold hands on his testicles. He looked at the posters around the room because he was embarrassed by the exam. It made him feel vulnerable.

"All done," said Dr. Brenner.

"So?"

The doctor sat back down in his chair and folded his hands. "All right, here's the deal. You're a bit late to the puberty party. But I do see signs that it's started for you, and I think the hair and the growth spurt will come soon. If you were seventeen, that'd be a different story, but you're fourteen. Listen, I don't recommend hormone shots."

A look of relief came across Matt's face.

"Should I invite your dad back in?"

Matt nodded, and Dr. Brenner ushered Matt's dad back into the room.

"What's the diagnosis, doc? When do we start?"

"Matt's exam came out normal. It's still too early for hormones."

Matt's dad looked disappointed.

"There's no sense in interfering with Matt's natural growth processes."

"But he could be a great basketball player if he were taller."

"Not everyone's supposed to be tall, Mr. Stevens, and not everyone's supposed to play basketball."

Sitting in that clean, well-lighted place, Matt had a thought that surprised him. He didn't have to play basketball. Hell, he didn't even have to watch basketball or pretend to like it for his father's sake. He could ignore him. His dad was living vicariously through him, and Matt had other ideas about how to live his life.

In the parking lot, he decided to stand up for himself. He was shaking because he'd never done it before. He mustered his courage and told his dad, "I want to quit basketball." His dad merely nodded. The ride home was tense.

⊞

Matt's armpits flourished when he turned fifteen. Puberty ceased to be a source of worry. It was actually more of a chore. Three times a week, he had to shave his scraggly mustache and shoddy excuse for a beard. He grew wiry, itchy pubes. He got erections for no apparent reason and had to hide them with books and backpacks. He shot up six inches, and for a while his voice squeaked, but then it mellowed into something low and soothing.

By that time, he had picked up the clarinet. As he got taller, he developed a greater lung capacity. He got bored with the regular clarinet and switched over to bass clarinet. In the comfort of his bedroom, he practiced for hours while his dad watched sports downstairs. He joined the pep band, and when the varsity hoops squad lost game after game during his senior year, he laughed at them and had a killer time in the bleachers. The bleachers, he decided, was the place to be.

7

Nditai's Initiation

Fiona Cresswell

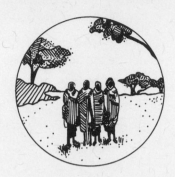

"Nditai's Initiation" describes a twelve-year-old girl's experience with circumcision in Tanzania. Female genital circumcision/female genital mutilation/female genital cutting has been performed as a cultural practice on over 130 million women worldwide, mainly on the African continent. A rite of passage from childhood to womanhood that takes place before a girl can be married, it is most commonly performed in early adolescence. It carries with it the risks of bleeding, infection, difficulties in childbirth, and psychological trauma. As a result, the World Health Organization has recommended the practice be stopped, and the Kenyan Government made it illegal in 2002. However, many cultures are reluctant to let go of this part of their heritage. The Maasai, for instance, are an indigenous seminomadic tribe in Kenya and Tanzania. The Maasai are divided into sections according to the geographic regions they inhabit. Each section's exposure to larger cities or towns and outside influences has influenced the ways in which they have merged traditional and modern ways of life. Many sections of Maasai are proud to maintain their traditional way of life and still practice female circumcision.

Nashami awoke to find her sister Nditai talking anxiously with their *yeyo* (mother). "I'm scared it will hurt and I'll cry in front of all our family," Nditai said.

Their yeyo replied, "This is a part of our culture and part of becoming a woman. My mother went through the Elatim [female circumcision ceremony], I went through this ceremony, and soon Nashami will also do the Elatim. Once you have been through the Elatim you will be ready to marry. No man will want you unless you are cut. I know you can do it, my girl." Nashami felt fear building in her stomach. She could imagine just how scared her sister felt too.

As well as fear, Nashami felt a sense of excitement that her beloved fourteen-year-old sister would finally become a woman, and for all the singing and dancing that would follow. The celebrations continued for two days after her brother's circumcision ceremony, known as the Eunoto. The community ate a great deal of meat slaughtered that day, and the dancing continued into the night.

No harm came to her brother Olemagu during his Eunoto. He didn't cry, and he became a warrior, Nashami thought, so why would Nditai have any problems? She felt better and put on her red woolen shawl and stepped out of their dark *inkajijik* (traditional house made from wooden poles, mud, grass, and cow dung) and into the bright light of the Mara plains, ready for the ceremony to begin.

Nashami, Nditai, and their yeyo joined the other girls who also would be circumcised outside their inkajijik. Nashami marveled at how pretty the girls looked with their shaven heads and beads of every color of the rainbow around their necks, wrists, and ankles. The invited practitioner, who would perform the cutting, and many other women, gathered around.

Nashami saw the knife called an *ormurunya* that was hanging in the leather belt of the practitioner and felt a knot of tension grow in her chest. She took Nditai's hand. Nashami felt her sister's hand sweating and squeezed it hard. Their yeyo made Nditai sit down and took hold of her arms from behind. The practitioner, an elderly woman from the community, lifted Nditai's *shuka* and wielded her knife. Nditai's body tensed as her clitoris was removed (it is believed this reduces sexual desire and promiscuity). Her brow poured with sweat and she collapsed back into her yeyo's arms.

Despite the obvious pain, Nditai did not scream or cry as she knew this would bring dishonor on their family. Nashami felt proud of her strong sister. Their mother then threw a bucket of ice-cold water over Nditai and applied a paste of cow dung and milk fat and a cowhide bandage to control the bleeding. Along with the other girls, Nditai stood up slowly, shaking as she put on a black shawl. Nashami painted her sister's face and placed her favorite bright blue and red beads round her neck.

The singing began and the women started their courting dancing. As is traditionally done, the warriors performed a dance, each taking turns to enter the song and jump as high as possible from a standing position, demonstrating their strength as warriors. The pitch of the haunting singing escalated higher and higher as each warrior's jumping increased in velocity, their words praising the courage of the girls and celebrating their coming of age. Nashami and Nditai's four brothers, their father, and the rest of the community joined the celebrations.

The sun reached its highest point in the sky, baking the dry brown earth, then set as a giant red ball over the plains. The dancing continued under the stars. Nashami, exhausted by the anxiety and the excitement of the day, retreated back to the inkajijik to lie down on her sleeping mat.

After some hours Nditai pushed her way through the reed door and collapsed in a ball onto her mat, crying and sweating. Nashami saw that her sister's black shawl was wet with blood and went to fetch their mother, who came and mopped Nditai's brow with a cool cloth and changed her bandage and shawl. "Go to sleep, girls, you have another long day ahead tomorrow."

During the night Nashami woke to hear Nditai mumbling in her sleep. She reached over to comfort her sister and found that she was burning hot with a fever. Despite the celebrations, the next day Nditai did not rise from her bed. Nashami took her a glass of milk fresh from her favorite cow and some cheese, but her sister refused to eat. Their mother brought the *laibon* (medicine man of the community) to their homestead, and he administered a medicine made from many local plants, which he kept in a small cowhide pouch. Mother was certain that it would make Nditai better.

The following morning Nditai's skin was still burning hot and she was delirious. Nashami was so worried about her sister's condition that she didn't sleep, and the minute she heard their cockerel crow she went to the home of the *legwenani* (leader of the community) and begged him to help Nditai. She knew their community was about a three-day walk from the nearest hospital and there was no way her sister could make it that far. The legwenani said their God Enkai had smiled on them because a community health worker from the nearest town would be visiting the community today and he would send her straight to their home.

Kazija, a community health worker trained by the African Medical and Research Foundation (AMREF), arrived within a few hours and examined Nditai. Kazija called Nditai's mother, father, and the community leader together.

"Nditai has an infection in the bloodstream and is very ill," she explained. "I have given her a shot of antibiotics, which is a medicine that may control her infection. But only time will tell if it's enough to save her life." Nashami's heart sank like a stone and she started to cry.

"The infection entered the bloodstream during Nditai's circumcision yesterday," Kazija explained. She had worked extensively with Maasai communities like Nditai's and knew that although circumcision was an accepted part of Maasai culture, removing part of the genitals in unclean conditions could cause serious bleeding and life-threatening infections. She checked Nditai's new, sterile bandage.

Kazija saw she had the attention of Nditati's family and the community leader, so she went on. "Some Maasai communities have now stopped practicing female circumcision due to the dangers involved, like what has happened with Nditai's infection. The World Health Organization has recommended the practice be stopped and several organizations are helping communities like yours to change the Elatim. This means that many communities still have the symbolic ceremony of the Elatim and give girls the rite of passage to become a woman. But they no longer perform any cutting."

Nditai's family listened intently to Kazija, but her yeyo looked at her with wide eyes, shocked that a woman could find a husband without circumcision. She had no idea that the cutting that was done to her, as it was to her mother and her mother's mother, could put her daughter's life in danger.

Nashami and her mother sat by Nditai's bed all night praying, fanning her to keep her cool, and giving her sips of water, sweet tea, and medicine. In the morning, much to Nashami's relief, Nditai sat up and asked for some milk. She showed signs of improvement each day until she was well enough to go out roaming in the maize fields as they were accustomed to do.

Kazija came again, with a team of health educators, a few weeks later and held a meeting with the elders and the women of the community to explain more about the risks of female circumcision. Nashami pleaded with her mother to be allowed to attend the meeting, but her yeyo said she was too young and she expected there would be disagreement during the meeting. Determined to know what was being said, Nashami and Nditai hid inside a baobab tree within earshot of the meeting.

After hearing more about the risks of Elatim from Kazija, the community leader began to speak. "Elatim is part of our history, something that has been passed down from our ancestors. What makes Maasai unique is the way we've held onto our heritage and our practices. We must cherish these and pass them down to our children. Outsiders will always expect us to take on their ideals, but we must resist."

His words were met with nods and sounds of approval. Next the girls heard a voice they recognized, their yeyo. "Our ancestors didn't have the knowledge that this practice could be so harmful. We now have that knowledge and we cannot ignore it. I nearly lost my daughter after her Elatim. We know what Kazija is saying is true. We must stop harming our precious daughters." Nashami had to bite her lip to stop herself from shouting in agreement. She was bursting with pride that her mother had spoken out.

After days of discussion and disagreement among the elders, it was decided that the Elatim ceremony would continue with joyful revelry and feasting but without any actual genital cutting being performed. Although many Maasai men still preferred circumcised women for marriage, the elders decided it was time to change their practice. Nashami was overjoyed that her sister was well again and that she and other girls in the community would never have to go through the pain and risks of a circumcision like her brave sister did.

8

Chris Not Christina

Judi Marcin

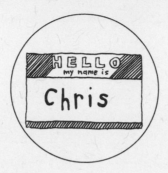

"Chris Not Christina" is the story of a young woman's quest to discover the person she truly is. Along the way, she questions her gender, her sexual orientation, and society's standards for both. Questioning one's gender and sexuality is a natural part of adolescence for many people and should be accepted as a natural part of growing up. Recognizing these feelings and exploring them is an extremely important part of living a healthy life. Through the process of realizing who she is and how she wants to live her life as an adult, Chris may do things she is not proud of but ultimately finds a way to be at peace with herself and the choices she has made. This is a story of being true to yourself and understanding the importance of friendship and filling your life with people who love you unconditionally, just the way you are.

Monday morning, Chris woke up to the alarm clock blaring the Violent Femmes. Without looking, she knew it was 6:53 a.m. Her clock was always set to some unexpected time. Never a 6:50 or 6:55, but something just a little off. And that was kind of how she always felt, a little off. She sat up in bed and pulled at her short, spiky platinum blonde hair and thought back to Saturday night. *It* had happened. *It* was real—regrettable but real—and now she had to figure out a way to make things better. Not just with her best friend Lauren but with herself.

She had felt so awful on Sunday that she spent the entire day in bed, claiming stomach flu. She was sure she could still smell the beer of Saturday night's party oozing from her pores. She remembered puking all over her bathroom that night, how the acid from her stomach burned her throat and mouth and how the cool tiled floor seemed like the best place in the world. And not only was there the spewing of Taco Bell that evening, but Chris distinctly recalled sharing some secrets with the senior class that she had intended to keep secret. She dreaded the idea of walking down the halls later that morning, listening for whispers of how a junior at a senior party had made a complete fool of herself or himself. What *would* they be saying?

Now more than ever, she wanted to be like everyone else. Blend in, not stick out. Be normal, whatever that was, and more than anything be sure of herself, who she was, and where she belonged. At least be like other girls, maybe just for a day. Her life would be so much easier. But she wasn't like other girls. She never had been, despite her mother's best efforts.

Her mother, Mary Beth Grace, born in Chicago but bred by the gentile South, was educated at an elite, all-girls boarding school in Charleston, South Carolina. She somehow managed to marry Chris's father, George Stuart, a physics professor. Chris was sure there must have been some sort of miscommunication along the way. Yes, her dad held some kind of patent, but no, not like the kind for the iPhone or Scotch tape. His had something to do with grain bins. So when her father got a job at a Big Ten university back in Illinois, her mother exchanged her glistening existence of dinner parties and beach houses for corn fields and cows as far as the eye could see.

When Chris was born, her mother gave her the most feminine and elegant name she could think of, Christina Louise. Her mother was fixated on the name, convinced it embodied grace, style, and poise, all the characteristics any young woman would want. Her mother did everything in her power to groom Chris to become the kind of woman who could marry a millionaire and look fabulous at cocktail parties. And looking fabulous meant dressing for the part. The pictures of Chris as a child that were plastered all over the house showed her dressed in every imaginable form of expensive fluff and every conceivable shade of pink. From the earliest infant sundress to the first-day-of-kindergarten matching skirt set, all pink—all the time.

As soon as she was old enough to understand her mother's visions, Chris tried to break out of the mold her mother had made for her. One time she ripped up a party dress so she could make a rope to scale down the banister without using the stairs. Another time she traded all of her Barbies for some of her best friend Herbie's GI Joes. Herbie wanted the Barbies for karate ninjas because they had such freakishly long legs. And Chris was happier with the GI Joes. They were much cooler and weren't pink. They really were camouflaged in the tall summer grass, which was the best way to sneak up on the karate ninjas in their evening gowns.

Chris always wondered why there had to be boy things and girl things. Couldn't there just be people things? she wondered. As she got older she understood that what a boy was and what a girl was seemed to be so clear to everyone but her. Maybe it was easier to conform even if it meant being someone you really weren't. And that brought her back to Saturday night. After years of trying to be different, she had been momentarily convinced that she desperately needed to fit in.

After endless summers with Herbie riding bikes and fishing, jumping ramps with skateboards, and learning to shoot a bow and arrow from her archery set, she had been told to grow up and stop acting like a boy, an idea she questioned every day. Someone had called her a tomboy once, as if he were insulting her. She didn't get it. So she was a girl who liked "boy" things—what was wrong with that? Why would that be an insult? She wished she could just be Chris, not a boy or a girl, but a person.

It was something like that she had shared at the party. She also had said something like maybe she wasn't really meant to grow up as a woman. Maybe she was born in the wrong body—and she was truly a boy. Maybe that was where she would fit best. And there was Lauren, her best friend, captain of her basketball team, and quite possibly the love of her life. But all this was confusing. If she liked girls but didn't want to dress like one or act like one, what did that mean? If she felt deep down that she wasn't one, was that even worse? And if she was in love with Lauren, was she gay? Her head was already pounding, and she hadn't even left the house yet.

Chris decided to miss first period. She didn't normally ditch school. She was an honor student and regularly on the dean's list for perfect attendance. But this was too important. She knew she needed to go to the clinic to correct what she could from Saturday night. She trusted Planned Parenthood. She had been there with Lauren to pick up birth-control pills and condoms, so she knew it was a safe space. People there had always answered Lauren's questions with kindness and without judgment. No question was too stupid or too immature. And maybe this day, they could answer her question, the ultimate question that was tugging at her soul: Am I pregnant? Chris was hopeful they would have the answers.

Saturday night had been more than sloppy, beer-laced kisses acting like truth serum. It had been more than wobbly words and unsteady, uncertain actions. *It* had happened, unplanned, unexpected. She had had sex with a boy, and not just any boy, but Kurt, Lauren's boyfriend. And not just any sex, but sex without a condom. She could hear what her mother would say if she were to find out. Things like *stupid, careless, foolish, you could ruin your life,* and *how could you*? It would be as if this had happened to her instead of Chris. But Chris was sure she wasn't going to hear any of those things. She had made a mistake and now was trying to correct it.

She didn't have an appointment. She hesitantly walked into the clinic and approached the receptionist.

"Hi, um. I might be pregnant." Chris could barely get the words out.

"OK, well, we can do a pregnancy test for you. How late are you?"

"Late. Um, I'm not sure what you mean."

"Well, the best time to take a pregnancy test is after you've missed a period. Before that, it might be too soon to tell."

Chris sighed and rubbed her forehead. She had no clue how any of this worked. I'm a high school junior, she thought. Aren't I supposed to know about pregnancy tests and how you take them? She wished she could talk this over with Lauren, but Lauren was last person she could tell right now. The receptionist seemed to pick up on her worry.

"Why don't I have you meet with one of our clinicians? Tell her what's going on and she can come up with a plan for you. How does that sound?"

Chris was near tears. She could only nod.

"OK, don't worry. Have a seat and someone will come get you soon."

Chris sat down. She was met with smiles and nods from other women waiting, women of all ages. As if they, too, understood how she was feeling.

The clinician called her back.

"Hi, I'm Carmen, I'm one of the nurse practitioners working here today. Why don't you start from the beginning and let me see how I can help."

Chris told her how she remembered it.

"I was at a party on Saturday and I was drinking beer. The problem is I had sex and I didn't mean to."

"Did someone force you to have sex?"

"No, nothing like that. I just wanted to prove to him I was girl, a real girl like Lauren. That I wasn't a weirdo."

"Why do you think you're a weirdo?" The nurse scooted her a chair a little closer to Chris's chair.

"I don't know if I want to be a girl . . . if I'm supposed to be a girl. I mean, I'm in love with a girl. What I mean is, I have no idea why I did what I did."

Carmen handed Chris some tissues. Chris closed her eyes tightly, trying to squeeze back her tears, but it didn't work.

"Chris, you're young and it's OK if you don't have all the answers. Sometimes as adults, we don't have all the answers. Gender identity, what gender we see ourselves as, can be kind of tricky. Not all of us are born in bodies that match how we feel. Sometimes we think we don't fit in because that's what society is saying. That this way or that way is normal. But you're human so that means life's messy. Who you are or who you love may not fit into a box of 'girl' or 'boy.' The most important thing is that you're safe, safe to live your life, and safe with the choices you make."

"Well, right now I'm not. What if I'm pregnant? We didn't use a condom. I had never had sex before that night."

"The best thing we can do for you today is emergency contraception, or 'the morning-after pill.' Have you heard about that?"

Chris shook her head. She wished Lauren were there.

"The morning-after pill is something you can take up to five days after having unprotected sex to make it less likely you'll get pregnant. It won't stop a pregnancy that's already started, but it can change when you release an egg so that at least you decrease your chance of getting pregnant when you haven't used protection. Taking a pregnancy test today won't help us know if you've gotten pregnant, but you should take one in two weeks. That will give us enough time to know if the emergency contraception worked."

Chris was so relieved she hugged Carmen.

"Thank you so much. Thank you."

"Do you have anyone you can talk to about all of this?"

"Lauren's my best friend, but I had sex with her boyfriend. I don't know if she'll ever talk to me again. She probably hates me."

"Remember, he didn't have to have to sex with you. That was a choice he made. So I think he and Lauren have some things to work out. You don't get to take all the blame here."

Chris was reassured. She trusted Carmen, so she asked one last question. "What about me being a guy? Am I like you said, someone born in a body that doesn't match how I feel?"

"That's something you have to figure out. Know that you can be attracted to men, women, or both. But how you see yourself is separate. Only you can determine the person you will become, but I know for a fact the only way you'll ever be happy in life is if you're true to yourself, not to your family or friends, but you. You have nothing to prove to anyone. Remember that."

Chris left the clinic knowing that at least she had done something to compensate for her lack of insight on Saturday night. Now she had to face Lauren. They had German together during fourth period, then lunch, and then they usually met up after school at the picnic tables in the quad. Since basketball season was over and graduation was around the corner, Chris knew she had little time left with Lauren. She would be going away to California for school. She might as well as be going to the moon.

Lauren came late to German and quickly left at the bell. Chris knew she knew, and it made her sick. She was the world's worst friend, and the most awful part about it was she didn't even like Kurt. They only ever spent time together because he hung out with Lauren. If any of the seniors had said anything else, it certainly wasn't clear to Chris. The day seemed to be clipping along as usual.

Lauren wasn't at lunch and Chris could barely stand the sight of food, so she headed out to the bleachers, thinking the old fresh-air-and-sunshine thing would make her feel better. And there was Lauren, sitting at the highest point of the football stands, writing in her journal.

Chris wanted to run up the steps but decided to be less impulsive and merely walk very quickly. She sat next to Lauren, who did not look up. Normally for Chris, being this close to Lauren caused rapid breathing and sweaty palms, but this day she tried to be thoughtful. She had to figure out how to convince Lauren to forgive her.

Without looking up, Lauren spoke. "You know I know, right?"

Chris nodded. But of course Lauren couldn't see that, so she cleared her throat. "Yeah. I figured."

"You also know you kissed me, right?"

Chris was certain she was going to throw up all over Lauren's Converse sneakers.

"Um, no, I don't remember that."

"Yeah, well you did, and you also told me you loved me. Is that true?"

Of course, you dummy, Chris thought. I mean, can't you tell?

Chris looked down and started messing with the string from her hoodie. "Yep, it is. Since freshman year."

"Well, I'm flattered."

"You don't think I'm strange?"

"Sure, you're strange. I'm strange. That's why we're friends."

"Lauren, listen, I am so sorry about Kurt. I don't know what I was doing. I don't care about him. I wanted to prove something. I wanted to feel normal. Now all I feel like is trash."

"I heard about everything you told Kurt, about boy and girl things and how society is messed up making people question who they really are. I actually blame him, not you. He totally took advantage of you and the situation. I'm sorry that happened."

Lauren closed her journal and looked out over the field. "I was writing Kurt a breakup note, trying to find just the right words. I realized there weren't any. He's a jerk. He betrayed me and took advantage of my best friend. So I decided on this."

"LOSER" was written in thoughtfully crafted block letters across the page.

Chris smiled with relief. "I thought you were never going to speak to me again."

Lauren looped her arm through Chris's arm. "You're still my best friend. I love you. Not the same way you love me, but I still want us to stay friends. I wish I could return all that love, but it's not how I'm made. But it's how you're made. I completely appreciate who you are—guy, girl, gay, whatever. We were friends before this and we're gonna keep being friends after."

Lauren rested her head against Chris's shoulder. Chris, at that moment, realized this was a friendship that was more important than any crush, any boyfriend or girlfriend, and it had the potential to withstand the distance that would eventually come between them.

9

Ariana's Decision

Kathy Wollner

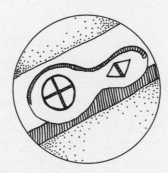

"Ariana's Decision" grapples with the issues of sexual initiation and teen pregnancy through the lens of a sixteen-year-old young woman. Ariana is charmed by the new kid in school and soon finds herself in an unexpected situation with him. When she learns she is pregnant, she is scared and turns to her mother for help. According to the Guttmacher Institute, by age nineteen, seven out of ten teens have had sex. Eighty-four percent of teens use contraception when they first have sex, most commonly condoms, but that means 16 percent do not. Nearly half of all pregnancies in the United States are unintended, meaning they are pregnancies that are mistimed or not wanted. In 2006, 42 percent of unintended pregnancies ended in abortion, while 48 percent ended in birth. In "Ariana's Decision," the course Ariana will take with her pregnancy is just one decision she makes. Through the challenges she faces, she emerges stronger, and we are confident she has the support to do whatever is right for her.

"Try it, mija, you'll like it," Ariana's grandmother said. Her mom gave her a look—furrowed brow, serious eyes. I'm watching you, it meant.

Ariana did not, in fact, like the cow tongue, but she made her grand-mother happy, smiling as she choked it down. It seemed worth it at the time, but the next morning, she felt awful. She felt nauseated and her head was spinning. She thought about staying home, but her mom had already left for work and she had so many absences as it was from stay-ing home with her brother or sister when they were sick. After making her way down the stairs to the kitchen, she ate her usual morning cereal before running out the door to catch the bus. She thought cereal might settle her stomach, but it only made her feel worse. Sitting on the bus, she felt the milk slosh back and forth in her stomach. Her friend Lisbeth had boarded a few blocks after her and was standing over her talking, but she wasn't really paying attention. She saw that they were approaching the bus stop closest to school and was envisioning the best path to take in order to vomit without anyone seeing her.

Ariana bolted off the bus. She had her eye on a potted plant that was just around the far side of the main steps. This early, there wouldn't be too many people around, she thought. She made it to the planter just in time as her whole bowl of cereal came up and out of her, onto the leaves and dirt. She could still feel pieces of cereal stuck in the back of her throat as she made her way up the steps and on to class.

That day she blamed the cow tongue. But two weeks later, throw-ing up again, she was pretty sure it wasn't food poisoning. Ariana looked in the mirror. Her eyes were red and her face was all splotchy. Glad I didn't put mascara on today, she thought. She pulled out her phone to check the time and decided she'd be better off waiting until the end of first period than heading back to class looking like this. This was the sec-ond week in a row she'd spent more mornings throwing up her breakfast than she'd spent in geometry class.

She'd only seen this happen on TV shows, and the women it hap-pened to usually weren't hiding in high school bathrooms. Pregnant? she thought. How could this happen to me?

The day before, she had talked herself into going to the store to buy a test, but once inside—and completely embarrassed—she learned they cost almost ten bucks. She didn't have that much cash. She'd have to scrape together lunch money for three days to pull that off. Unfortunately, she wasn't sure she needed a test to confirm her suspicion. Not only was she throwing up left and right, but her boobs hurt like crazy. She didn't have too much to go on, but since those were girl parts too, she didn't think it was a good sign.

When she had sex ed last year as freshman, it was pretty sparse on information. In addition to all the puberty stuff they'd already gotten in middle school, the basic gist of the two lectures was (1) do not have sex or (2) you'll end up pregnant, which will ruin your life and shame you forever, and/or (3) cause you to catch some terrible sexually transmitted infection. The health teacher showed them all sorts of hideous pictures of penises and vaginas with these diseases. No one wanted these diseases; the teacher seemed to consider the message delivered.

Ariana first met Chris a few months earlier, when he transferred to Cesar Chavez High School in the middle of the fall semester after his family moved from Texas. She rapidly developed a serious crush on him. He was good looking, but not too good looking in a way that would make him super popular and out of her league. Within two weeks he had displaced the previous class clown from his esteemed position as he brought the sort of drawings that were passed around classrooms to a whole other level. Some of them were mean, but as long as they weren't of Ariana, she didn't care. He was so dreamy.

"Gosh, Ariana, you sound ridiculous," Lisbeth said. "I mean, he's cute, but he's kind of a jerk. Didn't you see what he did to Max the other day?"

She had. Max was her neighbor, and while they weren't really friends anymore, Ariana still didn't like it when people picked on him. Chris had circulated a drawing of Max eating a stack of cheeseburgers. She'd seen Max's look of devastation when the picture got to him.

"Well, I'm sure Chris doesn't know how sensitive Max is," she said. "He was just trying to be funny."

That Friday was homecoming. Ariana wasn't planning on going, based on her general opinion that dances were lame, but she spent all week secretly hoping that Chris did not think dances were lame and would ask her to be his date. She knew this was farfetched, given that she hadn't had a conversation with him yet. It's only Monday, she thought, there's still time.

As luck would have it, she was paired with Chris for an activity in history class that afternoon. They had been learning about the civil rights movement and were assigned to read speeches and letters by Martin Luther King Jr. and Malcolm X the night before for homework. Now they were supposed to work together to come up with a list comparing and contrasting the ways the two leaders went about trying to change things.

"Hey," she said. "I'm Ariana," sitting down in the desk next to his.

"Right. Ms. Hughes just said that." He was drawing a figure with speech bubbles, but she couldn't make out if it was anyone she knew. She let the awkward silence hang in the air for what seemed like forever.

"So . . . are you going to the homecoming dance on Friday?" she asked nervously.

"God, no. Who would go to that?" She turned her head so he wouldn't see her blushing.

"I know, right?" Ariana said. "I totally agree, those dances are really awful, the worst."

He turned toward her and laughed. He narrowed his eyes as if sizing her up. "Well, if you're not going to the lame dance, I'm having a party over at my place since my parents gotta bounce back to Texas for the weekend. I got booze. You should come."

Ariana didn't know what to think. Wasn't he just laughing at me? she wondered. Does he really want me to come? Is this a date? How am I going to get permission to go to a party?

"I mean, unless your daddy won't let you go," Chris added snidely.

Ariana snapped to attention. "No, um, yeah, I can come. Cool." Despite her impulse to run out the classroom before she said something stupid, she did really want to complete this assignment. She didn't do all that reading last night for nothing.

"Want to start working on the assignment?" she said.

"I don't think you need my help." He had already moved onto a new drawing.

Friday night Ariana decided she was just going to tell her mom that she and Lisbeth were going to the homecoming dance. She figured it would buy her the right amount of time. She had made dinner for her brother and sister and was doing the dishes when her mom got home from work.

"Hey, Mom," she yelled over her shoulder. "Lisbeth and I are going to go over to the dance tonight. OK?"

"Sure, mija. Who's the lucky guy?"

"Nobody, Mom, the two of us are just going. Girls' night."

"But you don't have a dress!"

"It's fine, Mom. You don't have to wear a dress to dances anymore. No big deal, we're just going to hang out with friends."

"OK, then. Home by ten."

"But Mom, we're going to go get ice cream after, and it's—"

"Ten. You know the rules."

Relieved that her plan had worked, Ariana turned her attention to a much more complicated task: finding something to wear. After pulling apart the majority of her closet, she settled on a pair of dark jeans and a burgundy long-sleeved shirt. She put her hair up in a ponytail, took it down again, decided on a pair of earrings instead of a necklace, and grabbed a purse. She knew she should have called Lisbeth to come along, but she didn't want to risk her spoiling her chances with Chris. Ariana could tell she didn't like him.

When she arrived at Chris's house she could hear the music thumping from the sidewalk. She walked up to the door, unsure if she should knock or just walk in. After lingering for a few moments, she was saved the decision when a couple stumbled out the front door and almost knocked her over.

"Oh, hey, sorry about that. Go ahead in," said the girl. Ariana thought she recognized the girl from the senior class and remembered that Chris had an older sister. She entered the house, scanning the crowd for anyone who looked more familiar. Just as she stepped through the entrance, Chris spotted her.

"History class!" he said as he came down the stairs. "You came!"

Not quite what she was hoping for, but she'd take it. He gave her a sloppy half hug and led her to the kitchen.

"We got some vodka and juice. Help yourself!" he said, raising his own red plastic cup. Ariana waited until his back was turned to poor herself some juice without the vodka. She'd seen one too many uncles get drunk and was scared of what her mom would do if she saw her like that.

As the night went on, she thought things were going really well with Chris. He put his hand on her arm while he was telling her a story and even laughed at one of her jokes.

"Want to see my bedroom?" he said. He led her up the stairs and down the hall. Does this mean what I think it does? she thought. He closed the door behind him, sat down on the bed, and looked toward her. She stood off to the side, still holding onto her purse, not sure what to do.

"Well, come over here," he said. She went and sat on the bed next to him, he moved closer to her, and she felt the mattress sag. He put his arm around her shoulders and leaned in to kiss her. As they were making out, she kept thinking about the strong taste of alcohol on his breath and how he used too much tongue. His hands wandered under her shirt. As he started to unbutton her jeans, her hand moved to stop him. He looked at her, startled.

"Come on, you like me don't you?"

She didn't know what to say. She did. But she wasn't sure if she wanted this. She nodded. She didn't try to stop him after that.

It hurt a lot more than she thought it would, and it was over really fast. Chris flopped off of her. "Sweet. I'm gonna go grab another drink."

As Ariana got up to put her underwear and jeans back on, she saw the alarm clock next to the bed. Shoot, I'm gonna be late, she thought, brushing a tear from her face. She grabbed her purse from beside the bed and ran down the stairs and out the door.

Ariana found Chris at his locker that Monday. "Hey," she said. He turned around to face her. She lowered her voice. "Did you use a condom?"

"Hello to you too. What do you mean did I use a condom? You were there."

"I thought maybe I missed it," she said, unable to look him in the eye. She was mortified. She turned to walk away, but he grabbed her shoulder.

"Hey," his voice dropped softer, "what was with that blood? Were you on your period or somethin'?"

"No."

Understanding seemed to register on his face. "That was your first time?" he said disbelievingly.

"Yep," she said.

"Well then, don't worry. You can't get pregnant on the first time. Trust me," he said as he grabbed his books and took off.

He hadn't talked to her since that day by the lockers.

She racked her brain trying to remember the last time she'd had her period. Since she started having it when she was eleven, it never had happened every month like her mom told her it would. Sometimes it would wait two, even three months before it would start up again. That was fine with her. She hated dealing with the pads and the stained clothing; it was all a huge pain. Now she wanted it to show up. You thought you were pregnant? Ha! She'd laugh at herself. All just a big misunderstanding.

She ran into Lisbeth in the hallway before lunch. "Ari! What's with you lately? You're acting like a zombie or something." Ariana knew Lisbeth meant well, but she wasn't helping. She wasn't sure if she could trust her. What if she tells someone?

She pulled her into the corner, took a deep breath, then whispered, "I think I'm pregnant." Lisbeth let out a gasp.

"Shhh!" Ariana put her finger in front of her mouth and looked desperate. Maybe telling her friend wasn't the best idea.

"What are you gonna do?"

▩

Ariana's mother had always told her she didn't want her to end up like she had.

"Ari," she'd say, "now don't get me wrong, you're the best thing that ever happened to me." Ariana knew there was a "but" coming. "But I wish I hadn't been so young when I had you."

Ariana had heard this more than once. There was never a follow-up sentence, but her mother's message was clear. Don't do what I did. I expect more from you. You can do better for yourself.

Ariana was terrified of the anger—or worse, the disappointment— she would face from her mother if she told her. When she told her. She needed help and she didn't know who else to turn to.

On the bus ride home, she noticed a sign across from her that read "Pregnant? Need help?" The sign mentioned free pregnancy tests, but the woman on the sign looked so sad. That might be where I can go, Ariana thought. But she knew she'd have to tell her mom first.

▩

She waited until her siblings went to bed. Her mom was sitting on the couch watching TV, but she looked like she might be falling asleep. "Mom?"

Startled, her mom woke up. "Yeah, Ariana?"

Ariana sat in the La-Z-Boy opposite the couch. She knew what she needed to say, but she was having trouble getting the words out. "I . . ."

"What is it, mija?" her mom said, now looking worried.

"I think I'm pregnant."

Her mom put her head in her hands and was silent for what seemed like forever. When she did finally speak, it wasn't what Ariana expected.

"Mija, why didn't you tell me you were dating someone? We could've talked about this."

"It's not like that, Mom. It's not somebody. It's just . . ." She broke down in tears. Her mom came over to her and wrapped her up in a big hug. Ariana let go of the sobs she had been choking back all week. She cried for thinking Chris really liked her, for not using a condom when she knew better, for letting her mom down. She cried for not having come to her mom sooner. She had spent so much time feeling afraid.

"Well, we've got to go see the doctor and get you a test to make sure," her mom said into her ear.

"I saw a sign on the bus for a place," Ariana said. "It said they have free tests."

Her mom leaned back from the hug, a stern look on her face. "Ari, that's not a good place." She sighed. "They don't believe women have choices when they're pregnant. We'll go see someone at the clinic. They'll help us."

Ariana sat waiting for her name to be called, biting at her cuticles out of habit and nerves. She'd hadn't been to the doctor in years. While her siblings had the bad luck of many ear aches and sore throats, Ariana had always been healthy.

When her name was called, her stomach dropped.

The woman who had called her name ushered her to the back part of the clinic.

"Hi, Ariana. My name is Jessica, I'm a medical assistant working with the doctor today. Go ahead and put your things down in this room here. This is where you'll come back to after you go to the bathroom. We need a urine sample for the pregnancy test. Just pee into this plastic cup and place it in the marked container to your left as you come out."

Ariana filled the pee cup as directed and headed back to her designated room. There were posters on the walls with information on childhood vaccines and how to eat well. There was even a small bowl filled with condoms on the counter by the sink. For too long Ariana was left alone with her thoughts. *I know she's busy, but I wish she'd get here already,* she thought. Finally, there was a knock at the door.

"Yes?" Ariana replied.

The doctor entered the room. She didn't look like Ariana thought she would. She remembered doctors looking scary and kind of bossy, but this doctor looked like a normal person.

"Hi, Ariana. I'm Dr. Hernandez. How are you today?"

"Fine, thanks," she said. "You?"

"I'm just fine, thanks for asking. What can I help you with today?"

"I peed in the cup like she asked. I think I'm pregnant and I wanted to make sure, I guess. My mom said I should come here."

"Well, I'm glad you came. I'm sure you're anxious to hear the results of the pregnancy test, but while we're waiting on those, since I don't know you yet, I do have some questions I want to ask you. "

"OK," she said, trying her best to calm her nerves. The doctor asked her if she took any medicines or had any allergies and questioned her about any times she was sick. She went on to ask when she first started having her period, whether her periods were heavy, and if they came every month.

"It doesn't really come every month like my mom said it would. Sometimes it's gone for a while, or comes sooner than I think it's supposed to. Is that bad?"

"Not necessarily. A lot of women have what we call irregular periods in their teenage years after they first start menstruating. Often, it can be helpful to start a birth-control pill to help keep the hormones in balance to make your period more predictable and a bit lighter. Birth-control pills are used to prevent pregnancy, but can be used for just this reason too. But we can come back to that in a bit," she paused. "Now, Ariana, I'm going to go through a set of questions I ask all my patients, and especially those who come in for pregnancy tests."

Ariana nodded. "All right."

"Do you have sex with men, women, or both?"

"It just happened the one time." She started rambling. "I liked this guy, and I went to his party, and he brought me up to his room. He's not, like, my boyfriend or anything. God, he doesn't even talk to me." She let out a deep breath. She felt relieved to be able to tell the whole story. She felt comfortable with this doctor. "It was a big mistake. I wish I would have just really told him to stop." Tears streamed down her face. "I just wanted him to like me."

"Did he force you to have sex when you didn't want to?"

She shook her head. "No. I let him keep going. It's all my fault."

"It's not your fault. These things can be very confusing, especially at your age. But no one has the right to pressure you into anything you're not ready for. And if you say, 'No' or 'Stop' or 'I'm not ready,' you have the right to be listened to. I like to tell my patients that there's no right time to have sex, but there is usually a time that feels right for each person. When you feel comfortable and not afraid. When you don't feel like you're being pressured. When you're with someone you trust. This doesn't always mean someone you're in a relationship with, but with a person who respects you and makes you feel safe."

"I didn't really think about it like that," Ari said. "I just wanted him to like me, and since everyone else has sex, it didn't seem like such a big deal. Now I really wish I would have thought more. I didn't go there thinking that's what would happen. I don't know what I expected."

"Well, since we can't go back and undo things, we'll just have to move forward from here. How do you think you'll feel if your pregnancy test is positive?"

"Scared. I don't know what to do. I'm only sixteen! I'm not ready for a kid."

"OK. And how do you think you'll feel if it is negative?"

"Relieved. I'm just so overwhelmed."

Dr. Hernandez passed Ariana the tissue box. "I'm going to step out for a minute and get those results. I'll be right back."

When she came back in, Ariana couldn't tell from the doctor's face what the answer was. She sat down and said, very calmly, "The test is positive, which means you are pregnant."

Ariana's shoulders slumped and she hung her head. "I knew it."

"Would you like me to go over options for the pregnancy now or would you like some time to process first? I can fit you in for an appointment later this week if you'd like."

"I'm ready now," Ariana said. "I would have been more surprised if it was negative, I just hoped it would be."

"All right. There are three possible options for any pregnancy. I'm going to say them in no particular order. You can decide to continue the pregnancy and choose to parent, you can decide to continue the pregnancy and choose adoption, or you can decide not to continue the pregnancy and choose an abortion. I can help you work out the next steps for any of those options. If you want to continue the pregnancy, you would start with prenatal care. For now, that would mean coming to the clinic every month for a checkup to make sure the pregnancy is healthy. In that case, you could keep seeing me as your doctor. Prenatal care is totally covered under your medical card. If you want to end the pregnancy, I send all of my patients to a friend and colleague who works at a different clinic. She's a very good doctor. Unfortunately, your public insurance won't cover an abortion, but the people who work at her clinic often help women get outside money to help them. Do you have any questions?"

"I don't know what to do," Ariana said.

"That's OK. This isn't something you have to decide right now." Dr. Hernandez settled back in her chair. "Is there anyone here with you today?"

"My mom."

"Do you want me to have her come back? If you don't want her to know you're pregnant, that's your choice. But if you do, we can tell her together if you want."

"I want her to know," Ariana said without hesitation. "I can tell her the test was positive, but can you tell her those choices again?"

"No problem. I'll have Jessica call her back."

Her mom started crying when she heard the news. She gave Ariana another big hug.

Ariana felt relieved. "The doctor said she can tell you the choices too."

Dr. Hernandez explained the options to Ariana's mom and gave Ariana a packet of information to review. It had a worksheet that would help her work through her feelings and come to a decision about what she wanted to do. Ariana set up an appointment with the doctor for the next week so she could ask questions and maybe get her first exam. She left the clinic terrified of making a decision but relieved she would get to make it.

Hand in hand, Ariana and her mom walked from the clinic.

"I'm right here, mija. Whatever you decide, I'll be right here beside you."

10

My Body, My Self

Molly O'Brien and Aunchalee E. L. Palmquist

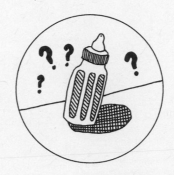

"My Body, My Self" introduces both the complexities of teenage pregnancy and childbirth and the important role that breastfeeding can play in caring for an infant. Teenage mothers struggle with many issues related to their changing bodies, changes that directly influence their self-esteem and identity. Pregnancy and breastfeeding in an unsupportive social and cultural context, such as in rural North Carolina, can be very challenging for teenage mothers, who worry about the stigma they may face from friends, family members, and society at large. Breasts are often seen as objects of a woman's sexuality, and for teenage mothers especially, feelings of embarrassment and shame often become barriers to seeking prenatal care or trying breastfeeding. However, breast milk remains the best nutrition for babies, particularly those who are preterm (born early). This story illustrates the importance of family and social support for teenage mothers and the unique challenges they face.

Casey woke up with a cramp in her neck, the gentle beep of Danny's heart monitor filling the room. He was fast asleep in his incubator, at the center of a dozen cords connected to machines with names she could not pronounce. She stood up from the blue vinyl recliner and stuck her hands in one of the incubator openings, delicately stroking her baby boy's tiny arms. She couldn't help but notice the contrast of her sparkly purple nail polish against his bluish veins that showed through his too-thin skin.

"Be OK, Peanut. Please just be OK." The nurse, Kellie, walked in with a clipboard to take notes on Danny and three other babies in the special care nursery.

"It's good that you talk to him, honey," the nurse encouraged. Casey pulled her arm away from her son. "Did you spend the night in that chair?"

"I just don't feel like going back up to my room. I wanna be here with him."

"I understand. Have your mama and daddy come to visit yet?"

"Not yet. We're still not really talkin'. I don't know. My friend Janelle is s'posed to be comin' to visit today after school."

Kellie nodded and peered in at Danny, taking some notes on her clipboard. "Well, on the bright side it looks like your baby boy is getting stronger."

Casey rubbed her eyes and pulled at her sweat shirt, instinctively placing her hand on her belly. "You wanna know somethin', Miss Kellie?"

"What honey?"

"I hated being pregnant. I mean, it wasn't so bad I guess, but it was just . . . my parents kicked me out, I had to go to a new school with a big ol' bump—I had no friends, no one to talk to." Casey didn't realize she was crying. "Now I guess . . . I don't know, I just wish he was still inside me. I wish I was still connected to him."

Casey buried her face in her hands, sobbing, and Kellie wrapped her arms around her, patting her back and saying, "It's all right, baby, it's all right."

Casey pushed away and shook her head. "No! It's not. What kind of mama am I to him? I'm fifteen, I'm homeless, he's got no daddy. I couldn't even keep him inside me a full nine months, I couldn't keep him safe."

Kellie reached into one of the pockets of her scrub shirt and pulled out a tissue. Just then the quietest whimper came from Danny in his incubator. Kellie smiled and said, "He heard you, Mama."

Casey reached her hand through an opening, gently running a finger up and down her son's belly.

"Have you been feeding him yourself? Like breastfeeding?"

Casey shook her head, not making eye contact. "They sent a lady in to talk to me right after he was born to show me how to use that pump thing. I tried once, but nothin' came out. It was weird." Casey paused before continuing. "Can't I just use formula?"

"The lady?"

"The breastfeeding lady. I don't remember her name."

"Oh, the lactation consultant."

"Yeah."

"Baby, it's *better* for him if you feed him your own milk. Look, are you gonna be here for a while?"

Casey shrugged. "Yeah, nowhere else to be."

"You stay put. I'm gonna send Tina up here. She's one of the LCs and she's gonna talk you through some stuff."

As Casey waited for Tina to arrive, she focused on the rise and fall of her new baby's chest and her mind began to wander. Soon her thoughts drifted back in time to eight months earlier.

It was one of the last warm days of the year, a Friday in October. Casey sat on the curb in front of her high school, waiting for her mother to pick her up. The school and the parking lot were abandoned. On Fridays, Casey usually stayed after school for student council meetings, but today she sat in one of the bathroom stalls. Mostly, she cried, but she also attempted to write letters to her parents and her boyfriend, Travis. She wasn't good with words, though, and eventually ripped up the letters and tossed them in the wastebin.

Casey's mother's white SUV came around the corner and pulled into the lot. Casey couldn't help but feeling like the "My Child Is an Honor Student" and "Jesus Is My Copilot" bumper stickers were accusing her of something.

"Hey, honey!" her mother greeted her as she got in the car. Casey managed a weak smile, not much else. They rode toward home in silence, the country music station doing all the talking.

"Mama, pull over."

"What?"

"Mama, pull over the car, please."

Her mother took the first turn into the Food Lion parking lot and looked at her daughter with concern. "What? You sick? What's the matter?"

Casey had a speech prepared, but instead she just broke down crying.

"Mama . . . I'm . . ."

"What? What's wrong? Tell me, baby." Her mother reached out and stroked Casey's hair lovingly, the way she had when Casey was small. Casey squeezed her eyes shut and pretended she was back in the bathroom at school, practicing what she was about to say.

"I'm pregnant. I'm pregnant, Mama." Casey opened her eyes as she felt her mother's hand pull away fast like she had touched something hot.

"What?" her mother demanded, her voice cold and winded. "No you're not," she said defiantly.

"Yes I am. I went to the clinic."

"You what?" her mother howled.

"Janelle took me to the free clinic after school yesterday."

"Are you kidding me? Is this a joke? Last week you're asking me to buy you fruit rolls, today you're telling me you've got yourself *pregnant*!"

Casey could only nod. It was here her mother snapped. She grabbed Casey's left hand hard and ripped the silver band off her ring finger—the purity ring her parents had given her when she was thirteen. Her mother held the ring inches from Casey's face and hissed, "Your father and I expected better from you. You were a good girl and you knew better. I can't even look at you now." In one swift motion, she rolled down the window, tossed the ring onto the pavement, and sped off toward home.

Telling her father was significantly worse. The three of them sat in the living room, Casey feeling like a ghost as her parents talked *about* her but not *to* her. She couldn't help but think that at least her mother hated her; her father was suddenly indifferent to her.

When he finally spoke to her, he simply said, "It's settled. You're going live with your maw maw in Ayden until you have it. Then you'll put it up for adoption." He spoke to her like a stranger; the man who had cheered the loudest at all of her soccer games and held her hand on the first day of kindergarten looked at her now like she was nothing.

Casey's daze was interrupted by a cheerful voice. "Hi, Casey, I'm Tina, one of the LCs. And is this Daniel?"

Casey nodded. "Danny, I'm calling him Danny."

"He's beautiful," Tina said. "He looks just like you!"

Cassie shrugged. "He kinda looks like my—his daddy. But it's nice of you to say."

"Kellie said he was born Tuesday?"

"Yeah, he was only thirty-four weeks."

"So he is just about three days old. I see here on his chart he's a little jaundiced. And you haven't been breastfeeding him at all?"

"No, he's been gettin' formula. But"—Casey paused and took in a deep breath—"I'm not trying to be rude or nothin', but it's sorta gross. My mama didn't with me and I just never thought I would."

"I understand why you might think that, honey, it's completely normal. But it's really not as bad as you might think. In fact, almost all the mothers I know say it's pretty wonderful. It's something special that only *you* can do for him."

Casey didn't know why, but she felt tears in her eyes.

"And because he is a little early," Tina continued, "there is nothing better for him right now than his mama's milk, which has all of the extra-good stuff he needs to get strong enough to go home."

Casey shrugged and sighed before she would allow the tears to fall. "I guess I'll try it."

"OK, sweetie, I'm going to get you to wash your hands real quick right over there and then we'll get started."

Casey walked to a sink on the other side of the ward and washed her hands while she watched Tina set up a small yellow contraption that reminded her of a lunchbox. It was attached by rubber tubes to two small baby bottles with suction cup lids. Casey sat back down in her recliner and let Tina pull the privacy screen around them.

"All right, Miss Casey, now I'm going get you to unbutton your gown for me and take off your bra."

"I'm not wearing one. They hurt."

"Your breasts hurt?"

"They feel like . . . I don't know, swelled up?"

"That's because you have so much milk, honey. Usually it'll dry up on its own because it's a supply-and-demand sort of thing, but right now your body knows it's got a growing little boy it wants to feed!"

Casey forced a smile.

"This is a breast pump," Tina said. "I know it looks a little scary, but it's easy enough to use. These two little suction cups go exactly where you think they might, so I'm going get you to put them on yourself and then we'll make sure they're the right size for you."

Once the cups were fitted and comfortable, Tina pushed a button on the yellow box, explaining that the pump would start in what was called "let down mode" and would then begin expressing the milk. Casey watched with trance-like fascination as her body, with the help of the breast pump, filled each of the small bottles in her hands. It was an odd sensation, there was no denying that, but the weirdness of it could hardly outweigh the relief.

When she was done, Tina helped Casey detached the suction cups and turn off the machine. She then showed Casey how to properly store the milk. Casey hadn't even noticed that Danny was squirming slightly in his incubator, and she realized she was grateful for the brief distraction.

"I think our little man might be hungry. You wanna try putting all that hard work to use?"

"I'm still not OK with holding him. I'm afraid I'll break him or something."

"Oh, sweetie!" Tina laughed, "I know he seems fragile, but you'd be surprised how tough babies are! Trust me, it'll be fine."

Casey felt herself smile for the first time in days. Tina poked her head out of the privacy curtain and peered around until she saw Kellie.

"Nurse Kellie, Miss Casey's going to try feeding. Would you help us get Danny out of the incubator?" Kellie came over and carefully examined Danny's vitals for a moment; then she began to gently unhook him from the monitors.

"All right, Casey, now we're going try something a little different. I'm not going to have you put your sweat shirt on just yet. It's actually better for him to be able to feel your skin, or what we call skin to skin."

"OK," Casey replied, eagerly reaching her arms out toward her boy. Despite sitting only feet away from him since his birth, this was the first time Casey felt a physical pull toward her son. She felt like a paper clip and he was a magnet. Kellie helped Casey get Danny nestled against her, although it seemed as though Danny's tiny head fit perfectly in the crook of Casey's arm and would have settled there naturally. Danny did look just like Travis. There was no denying that—from the head of dark-brown hair to the slightly furrowed brow—and it broke Casey's heart how beautiful he was. Tina handed the bottle of breast milk to Casey and showed her how to hold her son. Danny devoured the milk like he had never tasted anything so wonderful, and as he sucked at the bottle, he reach up a tiny hand and clasped it around his mother's pinky. Casey couldn't help but giggle with pride at his strength, and she didn't realize she was crying until a large, happy tear landed on her baby's shoulder.

Casey's health class covered human reproduction two weeks after she lost her virginity to Travis. All twenty of the people in her class sat there feeling mortified as Mr. Hargrove, the baseball coach, went on and on about child development, reproductive health, and breastfeeding. Casey and Janelle walked to lunch afterward, talking about this new information.

"I would never breastfeed my babies!" Janelle concluded emphatically. "My mama didn't with me and her mama didn't for her. It's trashy, walking around with your baby hanging off you like that just 'cause you can't afford formula or whatever."

"Yeah, it's gross. But apparently it's better for them or something," Casey offered.

"Nah, maybe it used to be but there's no way that's true, right? It's just nasty, end of story. I am never using my breasts to feed a baby, that's why God made bottles, thank you very much! And I can't stand it when I see someone breastfeeding their baby just any 'ol place. Like, don't just whip that thing out when other people are around. No one wants to look at that!"

The two girls were suddenly silent and locked eyes before dissolving into uncontrollable laughter.

Casey hadn't started showing until she was about five months along, and she was thankful for her maw maw's screened-in porch, where she could sit and read and manage to stay cool. It was around this time that Travis managed to come down to Ayden to visit her for the first time since she had told him about the pregnancy. Not unlike her own parents, Travis's mother was very religious and didn't like the idea of him constantly going to visit his "knocked-up" girlfriend. Fortunately, they managed to e-mail and talk on the phone a few times a week. Now it was Thanksgiving break and he had told his mother he was going to drive up to Raleigh to visit a friend at State.

Casey couldn't have pictured a more romantic reunion. Despite her swollen belly, Travis wrapped his arms around her and spun her around in a loving embrace. Casey had made sure to tell him to arrive while her maw maw was at her women's luncheon at the church so they could have some time alone together. She showed him around the house, the porch, the yard, and told him about all the books she had been reading, and he gave her updates on everyone back home that she hadn't already heard from Janelle. They had finally ended up sitting on her bed in the guest room.

"Baby, I missed you so much. Are you feeling all right?"

"I don't know. It's not real comfortable, I guess. It's hard to get used to seeing myself all fat. It's like a surprise whenever I look in the mirror."

"Well, I think you still look just as hot as ever," Travis said reassuringly as he leaned in for a kiss. As they were lying side by side on her bed together, Casey couldn't help but feel that things were finally close to normal. But then Travis pushed away from her slightly and said, "I guess the one good thing is I don't have to wear a condom now."

"What?" Casey asked, tilting her head to the side, certain she had misunderstood.

"Well, you're not gonna get pregnant again if you're already pregnant!" He laughed, leaning back in to pick up where they had left off. Now it was her turn to pull away.

"Wait, Travis, I don't want to have sex."

"No, it's all right, I Googled it. The baby can't feel nothing—so it's okay."

"No, Travis, I know I *can*. I said I don't *wanna*."

He sat up on the bed and stared down at her indignantly. "Then what the hell did I come out here for, Casey? I mean damn, I haven't seen you in almost six months and now you say you don't want to be with me!"

"I didn't! I do want to be with you. I love you. But I just don't feel like myself and I don't want to have sex when I feel like this."

Travis shook his head. "Look, I get that you feel like you're all fat or whatever. But you're still you. You're still *my* girlfriend and I should still be able to be with you like this. If you don't feel like being with me, how in the hell are we gonna raise a baby together?"

"That's not fair!"

"*This* isn't fair! You think I'm ready to deal with this? You know what? It was a stupid idea to come here. I need to leave."

And he did. He left her sitting there, half-dressed on the guest bed in her maw maw's house, crying. Casey felt so confused. She walked over to the hallway mirror, staring at her watermelon-sized belly. "I used to be pretty," she murmured. "Now look at me. Ughhhhhh," she growled in disgust.

Casey and Travis hadn't spoken since that day. Janelle called him the day Danny was born, but Travis never came to the hospital to visit. "Good riddance," said Janelle, "he's such a jerk. You're both better off without him." Casey knew she was right, but it still hurt to think about it.

After Danny finished the bottle of breast milk, he fell asleep on Casey, his bare chest against hers, the two of them covered in a blanket. Casey realized this was the best she had felt since his birth. Getting some of the milk out of her had been a relief, but feeling his skin against hers had done her just as much good as it had him. Tina had said that was something called "kangaroo care," meaning it was good for babies to know the feeling of being nestled right up against their mamas. Casey couldn't help but laugh as she imagined herself as a kangaroo, carrying Danny around in her pouch rather than having to sit next to his incubator.

Around dinnertime, Casey got another big surprise. Her mother and father arrived. Her mother was carrying a small blue gift bag; her father was still in his work clothes.

"Hi," her mother greeted her. But there was something like embarrassment in her voice.

"What are y'all doing here?" Casey jumped to her feet, not managing to mask her surprise.

"We just—your maw maw told us you were rushed to the ER. We were worried sick about you. How are you?" Casey could barely breathe as her mama squeezed her.

"Oh, just look at him. He is *beautiful*!" Casey's mother beamed as tears of grandma joy flowed down her cheeks. She reached for her husband. Casey's dad looked at Danny and began shaking as he wept.

"He's doing better, getting stronger every day."

"He is just precious. And how are you feeling, darlin'?"

Casey didn't know what to say. This was the most the three of them had spoken in months. "I'm doing all right, a little tired and sore, but all right."

"What's that?" her mother asked, pointing to the yellow breast pump next to Casey's chair.

"It's a breast pump. I'm going to try breastfeeding him."

Casey's dad cleared his throat. "I'm—coffee . . . uh, I'm gonna go get coffee," he said before nearly running out of the room. Casey's mother grabbed one of the other chairs and pulled it over.

"When did you decide to do that?" she asked, her voice surprisingly calm.

"This morning. The lactation specialist came up and helped me. I've pumped twice today—you're supposed to do it every three hours—but I think I might try to get him to actually breastfeed instead of use the bottle, when he gets a little stronger. And before you start about how it's trashy and you didn't do it I just . . ." Casey hadn't realized how defensive she sounded until her mother held up a hand for her to settle down.

"Just give me a minute before you start getting mad at me. I don't think it's trashy. Honestly, I think it's good. Did you know I wanted to breastfeed you?"

"What?"

"That's right. Your Nana Ruth and Aunt Jill finally talked me out of it. Convinced me that your daddy made enough money we should just buy formula, and I just listened to them."

"You never told me that."

"I didn't think it was something you would need to know when you were fifteen."

"I know," Casey whispered. "I know I disappointed you."

"Casey Beth, I didn't come here to fight with you. Your daddy and I haven't slept in months. We *love* you. You know that, right? We love you and we don't want you and this baby to grow up hating us or thinking we don't want you."

"You kicked me out, Mama." They were both crying now.

"We were angry! We were scared and we didn't know what to do."

"Neither did I. I was scared too!"

"I'm so sorry, baby girl. Listen to me. We talked this through and we want to support you. We think it would be all right if you moved back home." This was the last thing Casey had been expecting.

Just then, Kellie came into the room. "Hey y'all, visiting hours are over now. Baby boy needs to rest, and so does his mama."

"Mama, I love you," Casey said. "I love you and Daddy. I want you to know that. He—we—will need you." Her father came walking up then, two cups of coffee in hand.

Her mother nodded. "I love you very much, Casey. And I'm proud of you. You let us know if you need anything." She stood up to hug them good-bye.

Her father wrapped his arms around her. Casey couldn't remember the last time her daddy had hugged her like this. "You're always my little girl," he whispered in her ear. Casey couldn't help but cry.

Two months later Danny was able to leave the hospital. He was almost a whopping ten pounds. Getting him to latch on had been a challenge, with him being used to bottle nipples, but Tina had showed Casey how to use nipple shields to sort of "trick" him into taking her breast instead of a bottle, and after a while he got the hang of it even without the shields.

Casey started working part-time as a cashier at the McDonald's after her summer school classes and on the weekends and found she actually really liked it. It was a blessing to have her mama watch Danny while she was away. Casey was determined to finish school so she could get a good job that would support her and her son. She thought maybe she could even try going to college and becoming a baby nurse like Kellie.

At her last checkup, her doctor congratulated her on taking to breastfeeding so well. "I know it's tough," the doctor said, "being a mama at fifteen. But I'll tell you, I've had mothers in here in their thirties who don't take to breastfeeding the way you have!"

Casey couldn't help but feel proud. "I thought it would be weird, but honestly I love it! It's like having a connection with him still even though he's not inside me anymore. I don't feel like I'm taking care of him if I'm not breastfeeding him."

❖

Before she was discharged from the hospital, Tina gave Casey information on a breastfeeding support group for teen moms. "I think you will find it really nice to have other young mamas to talk to," Tina said. Casey stared at the card with the support group information on it for months before finally mustering the courage to go.

She and Danny walked into a room full of mamas and babies, some fussing, some giggling, and others sleeping. She couldn't believe there were so many other mothers her age who were also breastfeeding.

Once everyone was settled, one by one each mother introduced herself to the group. Finally, it was Casey's turn. She could feel her cheeks grow red as her heart began to race. She smiled nervously.

"Hi, I'm Casey. I'm fifteen years old. This is my baby boy, Danny. He turned eight months last Tuesday. I never planned to be a breastfeeding mama. I thought it was kind of trashy and strange. But then, I had Danny. He came six weeks early and he was sick—spent a few weeks in the special care nursery—and the thing that was going to help him get better was my milk. It wasn't easy, that's for sure. When he was born, I didn't know anything about being a mama. But breastfeeding was one thing I could do for him that no one else could do. I got so many things wrong in this life and never thought I could be the kind of mama my baby boy deserves. But all that changed when I was able to breastfeed him. It's like, I can't believe my body can do this! It's truly amazing. I may be young, but I am still his mama. When I'm feeding him, I feel like I'm a *good* mama. He's happy, and I'm happy. And at the end of the day, that's what matters most to me."

Texas Freedom Network
Kathy Wollner

Texas Freedom Network (TFN) is an organization that works on education and advocacy in defense of religious freedom, individual liberties, and science. *Advocacy* is working to make change in a way that supports your mission or goal. Related to health education, TFN works with parents, students, and public health advocates to help them improve sex education in Texas.

Abstinence-only sex education is the only form of sex education supported by state policy makers in Texas. That means students learn about abstinence—not having sex until marriage—but don't learn about other ways to prevent pregnancy and sexually transmitted infections (STIs), such as birth control and condom use. Even though many studies have shown that this method of sex education is not effective, meaning it doesn't keep young people from becoming pregnant or getting STIs, research by the TFN Education Fund has shown that most schools in Texas have strict abstinence-only-until-marriage policies on sex education. Unfortunately, Texas has one of the highest teen birthrates in the nation.

In 2004, the State Board of Education (SBOE) in Texas adopted new health textbooks that didn't include information about contraception and STI prevention, even though 90 percent of Texans support teaching students about these methods in addition to abstinence. TFN rallied sixty partners in its Protect Our Kids campaign, which called on publishers to revise their textbooks to include that critical information before the SBOE adopted them for use.

While abstinence-only education remains the most common approach in Texas schools, in recent years, there has been an increase in the number of school districts that have decided to include at least basic information about contraception (called abstinence-plus sex education). In the 2010–2011 school year, just over 25 percent of districts reported using abstinence–plus sex education programs—up from just 3.6 percent of districts in 2007–2008.

It is extremely important to have strong advocates to support good health education policies in the face of decision makers who deny young people the information they need to take care of themselves and stay healthy. TFN works with young people to place them at the center of advocacy in support of better, more comprehensive sex education in Texas.

DISCUSSION QUESTIONS

- What type of sex education do you have at your school? Is there anything that you didn't learn in sex education that you wished you had?
- How do you get information about sex if not from school?
- What are the policies in place in your state around sex education?
- Find an organization that is working to create good health education policy in your state. How can you get involved in its work?
- If there isn't an organization in your state or community, how could you and your classmates advocate for comprehensive sex education?

This section's information has been adapted from Texas Freedom Network's website. To learn more about Texas Freedom Network and to get involved in its advocacy efforts, visit www.tfn.org.

Section III

Mental Health

There is no health without mental health. This is a cry shared around the world by many activists, clinicians, and patients. Mental illness afflicts a large number of people and can be manageable with the correct treatment and social support. Mental illnesses are medical conditions that affect a person's thinking, feeling, mood, and ability to relate to others and function in their daily lives. Mental illnesses include conditions such as major depression, schizophrenia, bipolar disorder, obsessive compulsive disorder (OCD), panic disorder, post-traumatic stress disorder (PTSD), and borderline personality disorder. Many of these conditions are treatable, just as kidney disease, for instance, is treatable; however, in the case of mental illness, it is the brain, not the body, that needs treatment.

No health without mental health also means that people struggle with physical and mental health problems at the same time. People with long-term physical illnesses, such as diabetes, cancer, or HIV/AIDS, often face common mental disorders, including depression, anxiety, PTSD, and substance abuse or addiction. For example, someone with diabetes might also struggle with depression, and these two diseases can negatively impact each other. Some physical illnesses, such as fibromyalgia and irritable bowel syndrome, also are related to mental health problems.

The experiences that individuals have in life play a role in mental health. In some cases, stressful life experiences, such as childhood abuse or neglect or negative social relationships, can contribute to the onset of mental illness. For example, if someone is sexually abused at a young age and lives with that experience to adulthood, negative feelings associated with that experience can affect her or his mental and physical health. The young person also may find it difficult to form relationships with people, especially if the abuser was a family member or friend. Mental health problems that stem from such experiences are most severe if left untreated.

Poverty can make it difficult for people to be diagnosed with and then treated for a mental illness. Someone without health insurance in the United States would have difficulty both having a mental illness diagnosed and having it treated. In addition, not all health insurance plans cover mental health treatment, so even more people have trouble getting care. Whether or not a person gets treatment greatly affects his or her quality of life.

Treatment for mental illness often includes medicine and therapy. Many mental illnesses result from an imbalance of neurotransmitters in the brain, which are chemicals that affect mood, emotions, and reactions to experiences. Mental illnesses such as schizophrenia or bipolar disorder can be treated with medication to help balance these neurotransmitters. Depression and anxiety can be treated by a combination of medications and counseling, but in many cases people improve with one of these two therapies. Psychotherapy and other forms of counseling enable people to talk through their problems and address experiences that are or have been difficult for them. Other therapies for psychological problems include acupuncture, yoga, meditation, and support groups.

Social stress, which encompasses things such as bullying, poor self-esteem, and difficult relationships, plays an important role in people's mental health. Lack of social support can be difficult to measure, but one key way to measure mental health as a community health problem is to evaluate the number of suicides that occur among certain groups. Risk factors for suicide include mental illness, poor social support, access to deadly means (like a gun or poison), and substance use. While social support influences quality of life and illness management for people with mental illness, mental illness itself can also have social consequences. People with depression or anxiety may withdraw from society and have a more difficult time with friends and family members. In addition, adults with mental health problems can have trouble keeping a job, which can influence a family's ability to pay their bills. Thus family and friends who care about people with mental illness are affected too.

This section describes how social and cultural factors shape people's mental health and how people cope with mental illness. We begin the section with a story of schizophrenia, as a young man discovers his severe mental illness and learns how to live a normal life in "The Ties that Bind." We then turn to more common mental illnesses, such as depression and PTSD. "Chantalle's Secret" describes a young Haitian woman struggling with depression and contemplating suicide as a result of a difficult living situation. In "A Homecoming," Luke's father grapples with his PTSD upon returning from military service overseas, where he experienced several traumatic events associated with war. Finally, "Tenzin's Dream" describes how Tibetan exiles living in India cope with political violence.

As you read through this section, consider the following:

- What are the different types of mental illnesses that are common in your community?

- What are the different factors that contribute to mental illnesses? What role do friends and family play for someone with a mental illness?

- Mental illness is a common problem and should be recognized and treated. It's important that you seek support from your school counselor or an adult if you have been feeling down, have lost interest in things you used to find exciting or fun, have experienced changes in your appetite or sleep pattern, feel you have low energy or can't concentrate on anything, and/or think about hurting yourself or have thoughts that the world might be better without you. These are some of the symptoms of depression, and if you feel them, you should find a counselor with whom you can speak.

11

The Ties That Bind

Neely Myers

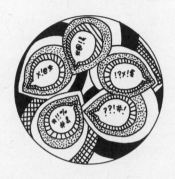

"The Ties that Bind" illustrates the experiences of two people living with a psychotic disorder. Psychotic disorders, such as schizophrenia, are very puzzling. They are characterized by intense experiences that come and go: delusions, or believing something no one else believes, like "aliens are controlling my mind"; paranoia, or thinking, for example, that someone is after you; thought disorders, or not being able to communicate your thoughts to others in a way that makes sense; and hallucinations, or hearing voices that no one else hears or seeing things that no one else sees. Some research suggests that psychotic disorders may be genetic; others believe that they have much to do with social context. The most recent explanation suggests that people who have a genetic predisposition to a psychotic disorder and also have stressful childhood experiences and use mind-altering substances like marijuana may be more prone to develop a psychotic disorder in young adulthood. Noah's story speaks to all of these possibilities while also helping us to consider what is at stake for individuals who have these unusual experiences and what they can do to work on "recovery," or finding a life that is meaningful for them in spite of their psychiatric disability.

One afternoon, after playing basketball at a friend's house, Noah came home from school to find an uneasy silence in his house. His little brother was nowhere to be seen. He wondered what had happened but had a strong feeling that it had something to do with Papa.

Papa stayed up most nights, poring over books in his study. Noah lay quietly on the floor outside the door reading his own books by the silver light seeping through the door, which Papa always left slightly ajar. Sometimes Papa would catch him out there and invite him in. He would curl up next to his father in his giant reading chair and they would read. Other times, Noah shrank into the shadows as he heard his father slamming books on his desk, crumpling papers, and ranting at something unseen. He knew that something troubled his father so profoundly that he stayed up most of the night, unable to rest until the solution had been found.

Noah and his father were both smart. Noah was in the gifted classes at his school, and his father encouraged him to read and pursue a good education. But when he told him why, Noah felt confused.

Noah's father warned him that there were people plotting against them, racist people. He told him that the world was full of people who could put thoughts in other people's heads. Noah was not sure what he thought of Papa's idea. He had never noticed anyone putting any thoughts in his head. Sometimes he came up with a new idea, but Noah was sure that was different. Papa said he could feel the thoughts coming from others. This made no sense to Noah.

On this particular afternoon, when Noah came through the front door, Papa, his tie askew, sat on the couch smoking a pipe and drinking a ginger ale on ice with a red plastic straw—his favorite. When Noah walked in, he smiled at him and patted the couch.

"Come sit with me, Noah," he said.

Noah's mother hovered in the doorway, looking worried. His little brother hid behind her dress. Even though the light was dim, Noah could see that Mama's face was blotchy from crying.

"Noah, go do your homework," she said, but he ignored her. He loved the smell of his father's pipe. He dropped his bag, took off his shoes, and snuggled under his big arm.

His mother sighed and said she had to check on dinner. She receded into the kitchen and his little brother paddle-footed after her.

Noah relaxed further into his father's side, but after a minute, he was overcome by curiosity. "What happened?" he asked quietly.

Noah's father hugged him closer. "I left my job today," he said. "I retired, so to speak."

Noah sat straight.

"You did?" he said in surprise. Their family barely made ends meet, he knew, and both of his parents worked hard.

His father nodded.

"Why did you leave?" he asked.

"They were just too racist, Noah," his father said. "They kept putting really evil thoughts in my head, and it is getting harder to fight them off."

"What kind of thoughts?" Noah asked.

"Really terrible thoughts. They are really good at it," his father said, a note of awe in his voice. "I couldn't take it anymore."

Noah sighed and snuggled in closer.

"What are you going to do now?" he asked.

"I am going to get my degree in psychology," Papa said cheerfully. "Wouldn't you be proud if your papa had a PhD? Then I could teach other people about all of these psychics who can put thoughts in our heads, so they will understand."

Noah felt very proud. Only really smart people had PhDs. People who had written books like the ones in papa's study. "Papa," he said, "are you going to be famous?"

"I don't know, Noah," he said, "but I think I will if I can prove that there are bad people out there trying to control our thoughts. Some people can't hear them, but some of us can. We need help. I want to learn how to help people."

"Wow," said Noah.

"Jake," Noah's mom said to his father, leaning wearily against the doorway. "You don't need a PhD, you need a doctor." Tears rolled down her cheeks, and Noah felt sorry for her. He did not understand why this bothered her so much. He knew his father was wrong too. Of course there weren't people who put thoughts in your head. But why should it upset her so much that his father thought so? Noah thought it would be very cool to have a papa with a PhD—a papa who wrote books.

Two years later, Noah sat in middle school trying to focus on the teacher. He felt very tired. His thoughts seemed garbled, and he was having trouble paying attention.

"Scratch, scratch," a sound went in his ears.

The sound was distracting, like when you listen to your heartbeat when you are trying to fall asleep and it keeps you awake. Noah had excellent grades, but he felt so disoriented, almost like there was someone trying to tell him something.

As time went on, Noah became more and more distracted and less able to concentrate. The air seemed to be glittering with patterns. People seemed to have rainbows around them. And there was someone trying to talk to him, he was sure of it. He could not quite hear them, though; perhaps they were just outside the door. He decided to take a bathroom pass from the teacher and check his locker in the hall.

There was nothing there.

After another week or so, he thought maybe he was just missing the voice from his locker. Maybe it moved every time he came out. He needed to catch it. He took out a bathroom pass in every class period. He was sure if he checked his locker at the right moment, he would know where the voice in his locker was coming from that he could hear in class. It did not occur to him at the time how odd this was—why would he be able to hear someone talking by his locker while he was in classes that were sometimes on another floor?

At night, he still read with his father in his study sometimes, and Noah still loved the smell of his pipe. He thought about telling his dad about the voice, but he was afraid of how he would react. Now that his father was in graduate school, he almost never slept, and the office was full of papers. Noah was not completely sure that Papa would listen to him even if he did tell him. He worked so hard on trying to figure out his theories about psychics that Noah often felt invisible.

His father paid the most attention when Noah asked him to teach him something. They had just made it through his father's old set of rust-colored encyclopedias, which Noah enjoyed. He decided to just keep quiet about the voice. Maybe it would go away.

But over time, the voice became more coherent until finally Noah could understand what it said. Once he could understand, it was hard not to listen. The voice had started off very nicely—it reminded him to do things, like sharpen his pencil, or raise his hand before asking a question. But then the voice became more complex. It was telling him really mean things about himself and the people around him. It was suggesting that he might want to hurt people because they did not really like him. The voice said people were just pretending to like him.

It was hard for Noah to look at people the same after that because the voice would be talking and telling him someone hated him while the person was trying to talk to him. It was very hard to listen to other people *and* the voice. And the voice really did not like it if he tried not to listen.

"Noah! Are you listening to me?" the voice would yell. Noah thought about asking the voice its name—it was about twenty-one years old, he thought, and a boy, but he just wanted the voice to go away, so he never answered him.

Noah began to think maybe his father would have some advice for him, but he was afraid his mother would find out. His mother often said that his father had schizophrenia and needed psychiatric treatment. For a long time, Noah had no idea what that meant, but then he and his father came across the word in the encyclopedias they were reading one afternoon. He remembered the day well.

"Schizophrenia," said Noah. His father lit his pipe and told him that the diagnosis was made up so that the psychics could cover up their secret government programs to control people's thoughts. Noah nodded and hurried on, but later on he looked it up at school. Words like "chronic," "severe," and "disorder" appeared with other words, like "breakdown of thought processes" and "paranoia." Noah felt dizzy, and he quickly put the book back on the shelf. He hoped no one had seen him reading about schizophrenia.

But the more the voice pressed in on him, the more Noah wanted advice. Papa heard voices too. Maybe he could help.

One night, late at night, when Noah was about sixteen, he could not sleep.

The voice kept talking to him, and he could hear it no matter how he tried to lie down. Exasperated, he decided to talk to Papa.

The house creaked underfoot as he crept up to his father's office door, which was closed. Noah thought this unusual, and he was not sure what to do. He stood there, debating.

He could not smell Papa's pipe.

He chewed his fingernails and rubbed his hands across his red hair. He stared at his freckled skin, picking at each freckle. But he really wanted advice from Papa, so he knocked on the door.

Softly at first. Then harder.

Noah pushed against the door, but it would not open.

"Papa!" he yelled, scared now, banging harder. "Papa! Papa!"

There was a loud crashing on the other side of the door and the door burst open in a cloud of papers. His father stood there, naked and bleary eyed, looking furious.

"What?" he hollered. "What do you want? What do you all want from me?"

Noah struggled for words.

"I was *asleep*! I am never asleep and *you* woke me up!" His father swung at him, and Noah stumbled backward. His father slammed the door.

Heart pounding, Noah turned to walk back toward his room. His mother stood in a dim circle of light at the bottom of the steps.

"Noah," she said hoarsely, "please don't bother your father at night anymore." She started to cry. "I don't want him to hurt you."

Noah thought that was a little dramatic. His father had never hurt anyone.

"It's all right," he said, wrapping his arms around his mother's shoulders. "I won't, I promise."

But Noah felt a great sense of loss; night was when he felt he could connect with his father. How would he tell him about the voices now?

Noah's mother and father started fighting frequently. His mother wanted his father to take school more seriously. It was taking much longer to get his PhD than she had planned, and she was working two jobs to cover their bills while he studied. But Papa was not attending classes regularly. He rarely showered or shaved. Sometimes he didn't even get dressed. He didn't have to go to work now, so he had no routine. He ate once a day, at most, and he rarely left the house.

"It's his schizophrenia," Noah heard his mother whispering on the telephone in the kitchen. "I don't know what to do; it's getting worse."

Other times, his mother would talk to a neighbor. "I know he needs medication, but he just won't go see a psychiatrist," she would say. "If you asked him, he would say everyone was a racist, and that's why he hasn't finished his degree."

Mama told Papa to just focus on getting his PhD, and then he could teach and everything would be fine. She cried when she said this, which Noah thought was annoying. Papa never cried. Noah was determined never to cry, either. His little brother cried, though. Noah didn't really know how to help him feel better, so he just hugged him when he seemed upset.

Along with most of his friends, Noah also started smoking weed. But unlike his friends, the marijuana pushed him further into the world of his voices. His perspective on his father changed, then, because he started sensing all sorts of messages from other people. He did not understand why, and he felt very disoriented. He enjoyed hanging out with people who were using drugs because everyone was a little disoriented and open to talking about altered states of consciousness without being too judgmental.

Meanwhile, Papa typed and typed, and the piles of paper grew and grew. He had typed thousands of pages. They swallowed his room and his desk. Noah knew his father's papers were all about psychology and psychic thought transmission. He had read some of them.

But Noah had a different perspective on his own voices.

At first he thought he was being manipulated by devils, not people with psychic powers. Then he was pretty sure the voices were coming from God. Thinking of them like that, he wasn't so afraid of them. If the voices were coming from God, not other people, then whatever they said had to be right. This helped Noah relax.

But Noah knew no one else would want to hear about his voices. He had watched his father try to explain his voices over the years to hundreds of people. They lived in the same house where his father grew up, and his father had known most of the neighbors his whole life. The neighbors had good reasons to believe him. He was a well-respected member of the community, a strong member of the church, a fine, upstanding citizen, a loving father, and a gentle husband. But neighbors, colleagues, and friends couldn't believe what he was saying, even when he wrote thousands of pages about the voices. He thought the PhD would help, but his professors did not like his theories, either.

Noah thought maybe Papa's inability to get anyone to listen to him made his paranoia that the government was persecuting him worse. Papa definitely had a lot of paranoid ideas. He thought other people were trying to make him become a murderer, or go to jail, or try to commit suicide near a cop so they would send him to a mental hospital. Papa was fighting everyone, it seemed, and he was not winning the battle. He struggled all the time.

❈

Noah went on to college, although he continued to live at home. One day, hanging out at his friends' apartment smoking marijuana, he tried to tell them what he was seeing.

"There is energy emanating from all of you," he told them, which made them all laugh, especially the girls. Noah liked the way one of them smiled at him, and he thought maybe she could help him.

"It's a little scary, though," he added, "because it seems like you're all trying to tell me to do something for you."

"Like what?" the cute girl asked with a naughty grin.

"Like maybe you are sending me a mind-to-mind message. Like to do something bad for you," he said.

"Like what, Noah?" she encouraged, thinking he was flirting with her.

"Like maybe you want me to kill someone for you, you know?"

Everyone stared at him.

Then they started laughing.

Noah tried to laugh, but he felt upset and awkward.

"That weed's making you way too paranoid, man," his best friend told him.

Over time, his friends told him he didn't do well when he used marijuana. They began to distance themselves from him, but Noah didn't mind. Noah lived in a huge city and it was easy to make new friends. Things were happening very fast, and anyway, it was hard to get to know any one person.

He dropped out of college, worked in a government office all day, and explored the club scene at night. He began to like the "rave" scene in particular. Raves were all-night dance parties. Their motto was very simple—to love one another and accept people as they were.

But one thing people at raves also did was take ecstasy, a powerful drug that caused them to feel, among many other things, overwhelming love and empathy for one another. Most people thought it also made it much easier to dance. Noah decided to try taking the drug.

He thought it might have been a "bad" pill, because after he took the ecstasy, unlike his friends, he started to get "messages." Now there were many voices instead of one. Celestial figures began to visit him: God,

Noah, Jesus, Abraham, and Mary. During these visits, God gave him the Torah, the Bible, and the Koran. He read all three. In them, he saw an all-embracing universe of many colors, a place where racism did not exist.

The messages were also very intense and commanding. Some of the messages convinced him that he was a famous rapper and producer. They told him that all he needed to do to let the world know was to lie down in a very public place and take off his pants. So he did.

And he was caught. He was arrested for indecent exposure and fired from work. Noah was devastated, and he tried to commit suicide. He felt that the voices left him no freedom to be who he wanted to be. They had too many demands. He could not separate fantasy from reality.

He was sent to a psychiatric hospital for the first time then, more than ten years after his symptoms began. When he first got there, they tied him to a bed and injected him with a medication that made him fall asleep. When he woke up, he felt very afraid.

When he was allowed to leave his room after a few days of good behavior, the people he saw frightened him more. Many were much older than him, slouched in chairs, staring off into space with dead expressions. It was straight out of a movie—burly orderlies dressed in white tying errant people to their beds. Noah was terrified to be one of them.

But he also had seen how people treated Papa for his wacky ideas, and he did not want to be treated the same. And the voices were so cruel, so loud, so insistent, that Noah was not sure how he was going to stay alive.

He couldn't remember telling the doctors about the voices, but they seemed to know about them. They kept asking him if he was still hearing them and they continued to inject him with medications. Noah felt very sluggish but also hopeful. He wondered if the doctors could stop the voices.

But the medications didn't stop Noah's voices.[*] He had been out of the hospital for several months when he finally realized that the

---

[*] Antipsychotic medications, in general, work for about one-third of the people with schizophrenia, meaning they completely silence the voices. They partially silence voices for another third and do not work at all for the other third.

medications weren't going to make the voices leave him completely alone. He was heartbroken. He tried to kill himself again.

The voices wanted him to stop taking his medications, and then when he did, they overwhelmed him with messages to kill himself. Now he wasn't sure if he had been taking the medications correctly the whole time. Maybe he had not been taking them well because every time he tried, the voices objected. Noah felt very confused.

He tried taking the medications all the time. At least they slowed the voices down a little. Unfortunately, they slowed Noah down as well. But it was harder to focus if the voices were really loud, so in some ways the medication seemed better than the voices.

Papa was strongly antimedication. He told Noah he just had to try harder to control the voices, but Noah was terrified of them. He was also terrified of becoming like Papa.

Several years passed, and by the time Noah was twenty-eight, he felt he had accumulated some wisdom. He had scars to show for each suicide attempt, but they were reminders for him to take care of himself, to try to be patient, and to give himself time to heal. When it came to healing, Noah had found a few things to be helpful.

Noah attended a peer-run service program. While definitions of *peer* vary, the people at Noah's program were people who had experienced serious mental illness, homelessness, substance abuse, and other hardships but then went on to lead lives similar to the life they might have been expected to have before they started having symptoms. Some peers even argued that their lives were much more interesting and fulfilling than any kind of life they might have lived before their symptoms started. Noah liked this message.

They recognize me for who I am, he thought. They know how it feels to be me, to walk in my shoes, and that gives me a lot of hope. They have been where I am, and now they are doing really well.

Noah's experience with his father had been really confusing, but the peer providers were different. They were much more empathic and did not judge him for taking medications. He wanted to help support that environment, to help contribute to the community. To build community, the peers often looked out for each other. If someone was absent for a day, for example, they might go out together and try to look for that person and encourage them to come back in and get support. They were willing to listen to each other as well, and provide support.

The peers worked hard to give back to others because they knew that helping others with their struggles helped those people to recover. People with serious mental illnesses can and do recover, but they need a lot of love and support. Before Noah looked for acceptance and support from people who were like him because they were using drugs. But drugs didn't help Noah at all. They made him much worse. So it was great for him, he felt, to find an accepting and sober community of new friends.

Noah told his peer group that he felt best when he was with people he loved. "My voices are quieter when I am with people I love because of God," he said at one group meeting. "When love is present, God is present, and God helps quiet the bad voices." Noah also found prayer to be very helpful. He liked going to synagogues, mosques, and cathedrals for services of all faiths because he did not believe in divisions by race or religion. He felt that there was one God willing to help him fight his devils. This gave him extra strength to try to build a more fulfilling life.

Noah was at the peer program several days each week. He came in the morning and stayed through the afternoon. The program was meant to be a one-stop shop so Noah could come there to see his psychiatrist too. His psychiatrist had also had psychotic experiences, and she took the same medications as Noah, so she understood the side effects of the medications. His therapist was also there. Noah even received a free lunch, assistance with employment, and group classes on skills such as how to act in a job interview at the peer program.

As he participated in the program, Noah realized that the best way to learn more about himself was to quit taking illegal drugs and focus on finding a meaningful job. He tried going back to college twice, but it was too much for him to handle. He couldn't decide which was worse, trying to take medications and learn or trying to learn while hearing loud voices. He decided instead to focus on improving his math skills so he could begin training as an electrician's apprentice. Focusing on work was very important for Noah because it made him feel that he had a purpose in life. At last life was going really well for Noah, and he was thankful for all of the people around him who helped him get there.

12
Chantalle's Secret

Ashley Hagaman

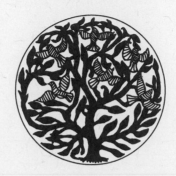

"Chantalle's Secret" discusses suicide, a complex, intimate, and far too common phenomenon. Worldwide, there are over one million deaths by suicide every year. Over 85 percent of these deaths occur within low- and middle-income countries, such as Haiti. Completed suicides are only a fraction of the problem as ten to twenty million individuals attempt suicide each year. Although suicide is frequently seen as a marker for mental illness, often social conditions, familial strife, or other social pressures drive an individual into the hopelessness that causes someone to consider suicide. Follow Chantalle through her journey and discover how community support, empowerment, and simple things such as empathic listening may help curb deaths from suicide.

"Goooaaall!" Étienne screamed over his opponents' cries. Running a winning lap, Étienne and his teammates laughed together as they saw the sun begin to set within the mountains of Haiti's Central Plateau, one of the world's poorest regions.

Étienne's family lived in a small town nestled in a mountainous landscape, many hours away from the bustle of Haiti's capital, Port-au-Prince. As the rest of the soccer team rushed to make it home before dark, Étienne realized it was too late to make his trip over the mountain to his parents' home. To be safe, he decided to instead spend the night at the *lakou* (home) of his older cousin, Chantalle. She had recently married and lived with her in-laws very close to the football field. It was much safer to stay with her than walk to his parent's lakou.

Étienne often stopped by Chantalle's home after school, or in the evenings when it was too late to walk down the mountain, and they were very close. Chantalle was the one who had taught him how to write the alphabet, how to dance the *konpa* (a traditional dancing style), and even to use a cell phone. Now that Étienne was thirteen years old, Chantalle had become a good friend that he could trust and confide in. Lately, though, Étienne had been noticing changes in his cousin, prompting him to visit her more often.

At nineteen years old, Chantalle spent long days cleaning the house, going to the market to sell the tobacco her mother-in-law and father-in-law cultivated, and caring for her two young babies. Her husband was always gone, working for another farmer. When no work could be found in the village, he would travel to the Dominican Republic to find farming work. Despite his hard work, he still made little money, forcing Chantalle to live in an overcrowded lakou with his parents.

Étienne knew Chantalle was frustrated, and lately he had often found his cousin crying. He usually tried to ask her questions or tell her stories to cheer her up, but most of the time her thoughts seemed far away.

Étienne entered Chantalle's home to the sound of a baby crying.

"Chantalle, your daughter is crying. I think she is hungry. Can we feed her?" Chantalle responded to his question with an empty stare. A few moments passed before she turned her head toward Étienne and nodded.

"Étienne, you are right. She is hungry. I haven't been able to buy food for her or her sister today. I had to give all my money to my mother-in-law. We live in her house, we must obey her rules. When she asks me for money, I must give it to her."

Étienne was aware of Chantalle's trouble with her mother-in-law.

Once he had stopped by the house only to hear her screaming at Chantalle and telling her she was worthless. Other days, he heard her scold Chantalle for not being able to support her children or build her own house. Chantalle's husband spent most days out looking for work, so the women and children were left alone most of the day.

Chantalle continued, "Last week, when my mother-in-law returned from getting water, I accidentally spilled the fresh water can as I took it off her head. I can understand why she was upset after walking two hours to get it. But she beat me. She beat me for an hour."

Étienne, unsure of what to say, leaned over and gave Chantalle a hug, squeezing her tight. Letting her go, he said, "You know how I come over here anytime?" Chantalle nodded. "That means you can come to my parents' house whenever you need to as well. And I promise I will always be there to give you a hug." Chantalle managed a little smile.

"Tomorrow," Étienne explained, "we'll see what food we can find for the babies. There's always something we can do." Chantalle sighed.

During the rainy season, life in the village changed. Every day around three o'clock, water was thrown down from the sky. It fell so hard, you couldn't see a thing. It washed away the roads, replacing them with pools of water and mud. In another nail-biting soccer game, Étienne and his friends once again forgot about the time. Before they knew it, their soccer ball was swimming in puddles of water and their clothes were completely soaked.

It was dark now, and Étienne sprinted to Chantalle's house. As he approached the front door, Étienne heard a strange sound. It was so faint and irregular that he could barely tell where it was coming from. He walked carefully around the back of the lakou. The noise began to grow stronger. He heard leaves rustling and a hacking noise as if someone was coughing under water. He saw a dark figure hanging from a tree fifty feet from the lakou. He carefully stepped closer and gasped: it was a human being, a person hanging from a rope around the neck.

Étienne ran to the tree faster than he had run in any football game. He yelled loudly for someone to come help. As he reached the body, hanging limp from the rope, he realized it was Chantalle.

Étienne desperately tried to lift her body weight so she'd stop choking, crying, "I'm here! I'm going to let you down!"

Responding to his cries, Chantalle's father-in-law raced to Étienne's side, cutting the rope with his machete. They lowered Chantalle's body to the ground

Many community members gathered to see what was happening. Whispers started to grow louder, each neighbor offering differing explanations of what might have been the cause of Chantalle's hanging.

"Do you think someone sent her a spirit? The spirit must have made her do it."

"How could we know? She never seemed to talk to anyone."

Another man offered his explanation. "She must have been *fou* [crazy], a normal healthy woman would never hang herself. Maybe that's why we stopped seeing her in town, because the family wanted to hide her illness."

"She must have stolen something . . ." Another woman chimed in, "A Haitian would never do something like this unless they disobeyed the law."

"No, it was because she stopped going to church. She doesn't remember the Bible; she has lost her way with God. She has sinned; she wouldn't have hung herself if she had gone to church. Only sinners kill themselves."

There were several nods and sounds of agreement from the growing crowd.

Étienne wasn't listening to the crowd. He knew Chantalle too well. He knew she couldn't possibly have done this to herself. They waited for what felt like hours for her to breathe. Chantalle finally coughed, and her body curled up into a ball. Étienne scooped her up and carried her into the lakou.

Étienne stayed by her side until morning. He couldn't sleep at all, and his mind wandered as he tried to identify the signs of Chantalle's unhappiness. His mind drifted to his last visit. He remembered her silence, her tears, and her sense of hopelessness. He remembered how she told him she felt like a burden on her family. Étienne desperately tried to configure the right thing to say to her when she woke up, but he felt so nervous and scared, fearing that no matter what he said, he could never help his cousin.

After many hours, Chantalle sat up. Her face was tired, with bruises beginning to appear where the rope had held her. Étienne waited for her to speak.

"Étienne, I can't go on struggling. I can't keep listening to my mother-in-law tell me how worthless I am. I feel hopeless. I can barely keep my daughters alive with the little money I have, and I can't send them to school. I have nothing left to live for."

Étienne sat silently for quite some time, trying to think of what to say. He wanted to be very careful with his words. "Chantalle, my cousin, I care about you. I love you. Your daughters . . . do you think they love you?"

"Yes, I know they love me." She smiled a little. "And I love them more than anything in the world."

"And your husband? Do you think he loves you?" Étienne asked.

"Of course he loves me. But I fear he might stop loving me because of my *mizè* [misery]. Why would he want to be around someone who doesn't even want to live? Why would he want to be around a failure? How can he love a woman who can't even make enough money to send her kids to school?"

Étienne let the silence speak as he gazed with caring and concern at his cousin. "Could you talk with him about how you're feeling? Could he understand? Your struggles are shared and they aren't all your fault. You can't blame yourself. That isn't fair to you. Do you think he might share some of your same worries?"

Chantalle nodded and turned her head away. "Even if he did understand, he is away working for weeks at a time. He is never home. It is too difficult to confide in him. Plus, he isn't here to take care of our children—he can't possibly understand how hard it is for me. The way my mother-in law looks at me, the way the other women in the community look at me. Like a weak and stupid woman."

"Do you think there might be someone else you would feel comfortable talking with? Someone who will listen no matter what you say and who won't judge you? I could be that person for you. I care about you, and I can help you through this difficult time."

"Thank you, Étienne. But no one can possibly understand how I am feeling. I am alone, I am poor, I am failing as a mother, as a wife, and as a daughter-in-law." Chantalle looked down at her hands and slowly began to weep.

"Chantalle, you're right. I can't possibly understand what it is you are going through. But I can promise you that I will always be here to support you. I know the reason your daughters love you is because you help them feel safe. You can offer them so much. Think of all the things you taught me!" Étienne stood up and started to konpa. Chantalle smiled, even though her tears.

Chantalle, her voice still quivering from crying, weakly said, "I will try, Étienne."

Chantalle's father-in-law walked in the room. Étienne curled in the corner, scared of what he might do.

"Chantalle," he said in a sharp, deep, and threatening voice, "you've shamed our family even more. It's upsetting enough that you are so poor; you can't even build your own house. Now we must all endure this embarrassment. You can't stay here any longer."

Chantalle's father-in-law towered over her, looking down at her with disgust. Étienne, still shaking, stood up quickly to face him. "She isn't an embarrassment. What's shameful is that her family cannot love her unconditionally. What's shameful is how much you make her endure, how much you torture her. She will come home with me, to my parents' home. Where her family loves her. We will treat her with the dignity she deserves." Étienne quickly grabbed Chantalle's things and gathered her children together before he ushered them to his parents' house

Weeks later, Chantalle began to gain back some of her confidence. Her husband had returned home, finding work with local farmers. He promised to stay by her side as long as she needed. Most of all, he promised to always love her.

After school one day, Étienne came home to find Chantalle sleeping again. Étienne woke her up; he had some ideas to share. With a nervous and cautious voice, Étienne began to bring up Chantalle's suicide attempt. "How are you feeling?"

Chantalle sat up, a bit groggy. "I still feel scared, Étienne. I still feel shameful. It's difficult to face my husband's family. It's difficult to feel hopeful with so much uncertainty."

"I know it must be tough," Étienne started. "Perhaps by speaking with others, you will remember how much love there is in the community. I heard on the radio that when you feel sad and hopeless, there's help in a town nearby. There's someone who works at a clinic there who is a psychologist. Her job is to speak with people who are having suicidal thoughts. She can help counsel you. There are many things the clinic can help you with as well. There may be a mama's club you can join to speak with other mothers who struggle with similar things as you. But I think the best thing we can do is to support you as a community. We can work together to watch your daughters when you need to work."

"Well," Chantalle began, "I am not sure about going to the psychologist. Étienne, I will remember when I am feeling overwhelmed and desperate that I can confide in you. I think right now I would like to speak with the priest. I think he may be most helpful to me right now. I feel comfortable with him."

"OK. I can walk with you to the church tomorrow." Étienne felt proud that he could help his cousin with something so serious.

"Thank you, Étienne, for your support," Chantalle said meekly.

Étienne smiled and quietly told her, "You are the bravest of us all."

13

A Homecoming

Erin P. Finley

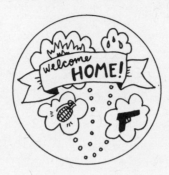

In "A Homecoming," an American boy struggles to make sense of why his father returns home changed after spending a year as a soldier in Iraq. Luke's father has post-traumatic stress disorder (PTSD), and Luke comes to understand the illness—and the impact it has on his entire family—as one consequence of going to war. It is important to understand that PTSD is a common psychological response to war and other traumas but those with PTSD can recover with proper treatment. Dealing with the effects of traumatic experiences is a common experience shared by many military families when family members return from war. Society often fails to acknowledge the impact of such trauma on the lives of people who have served and their families.

The night before Luke's father returned from a year in Iraq, Luke sat at the kitchen table and made a sign. He and his mom had been to the store earlier in the day and bought the biggest piece of poster board they could find. Luke wrote, "WELCOME HOME DAD" in black and red capital letters then glued a photo of a tank in one corner because his father drove a tank for the U.S. Army. He then stuck a picture of his little sister, Beth, and him in the other corner, with their arms waving. Across the bottom, he pasted pictures from Beth's fourth birthday party, from his own band recital the spring before, and from the weekend Mom took them to his uncle's farm—all things his father had missed while he was gone.

The next morning, Luke's mom rushed around the house cleaning up. She made Luke put his lizard Harry's terrarium back in his room. He had been keeping it in the kitchen because there was a big window there and Harry liked to lie on his rock in the sun. But Luke's mother said that having stuff laying around everywhere made the house look like a tornado had gone through it.

She finally decided the house looked as good as it was going to get and, turning to Luke, asked, "Would you sit and watch *Dora the Explorer* with Beth while I get ready?" Luke hated *Dora the Explorer*, but his mom looked so nervous that he said he would. She retreated into his parents' room, and he watched three episodes with Beth before his mom was ready.

She still looked nervous when she returned to the living room, but she had a dress on and smelled good. She put her lipstick on in front of the mirror by the door, and Beth, who was four, started begging to have some lipstick too. His mom looked at Beth blankly for a moment, then she smiled and leaned down to paint some bright pink on her lips. Luke went to his bedroom and grabbed the sign he had made.

They got into the car and drove over to the base, where there was a huge crowd of people in a parking lot over by the training field. They waited for what seemed like forever, Luke holding the sign in front of his chest. Then a big white school bus came around the corner, slowed to a halt, and parked as the crowd crushed in around it. The door slid open, and out came a woman and several men too tall or short or wide to be Luke's dad.

And then his mom, who was standing behind him holding Beth on her hip, suddenly yelled, "Joe! Honey!" and Luke saw his father take a step down off the bus, still wearing his gray-and-green battle dress uniform. He looked their way and his face lit up. In no time he had his arms wrapped around Mom and Beth and Luke and the sign all at once, and Luke was hugging him as hard as he could. He could barely breathe in the family hug. He could feel his mom shaking as she began to cry.

The first morning Luke's dad was home, he made Luke a bowl of Fruit Loops while his mom was still sleeping. Luke hadn't eaten Fruit Loops in months—he had a new favorite cereal with chocolate koalas in it. But he ate it anyway because it was nice to sit in the kitchen with his dad. His father asked him about school, and Luke told him it was going OK, although he didn't like Mr. Kerry, his math teacher.

After he was done with his cereal, Luke brought Harry out and showed him off, since he had only had him since the start of the school year. Dad hadn't seen the scar on Luke's elbow from when he careened his skateboard into the tree either, so he showed him that too.

Beth came into the kitchen and stood close to Luke, sleepy still and rubbing her eyes. She was shy with their dad. Luke thought that maybe she was so little when he left that she only half-remembered him. His dad looked at her for a minute then offered to get her some Fruit Loops. She shook her head and burrowed it into Luke's arm.

As good as it was to have his father home, Luke first got the sense that something was wrong a few days later. Luke had gone back to school after an extra couple of days home with his dad, who had a month on leave before going back to work on base. Luke's friend Jimmy came over after school, and they sat down in the living room in front of a new video game Jimmy had brought. It was a pretty good game and they were getting into it, flinging back and forth the worst insults they could think of at full volume.

Luke's dad had been sitting in the kitchen trying to read, and he came in suddenly and shouted, "Will you two knock it off?" before storming off down the hall. Jimmy and Luke both got very quiet, and when Luke glanced over at Jimmy, his eyes were wide.

Luke had never heard his dad yell like that. His mom was the one who was liable to get loud when she was mad. His dad was always calm, always the cool and steady one.

But after he got back from Iraq, his dad wasn't cool and steady. He was quick to get mad if he thought Beth and Luke were being too loud or not obeying their mom. The smallest things seemed to set him off. There were other things too. Jimmy and his father wanted to take the family to a basketball game, but Luke's father wouldn't go.

Luke couldn't believe it. "But Dad, it's the Spurs and the Knicks! And they're good seats! We used to go to games all the time!"

His father looked uncomfortable, then angry. "I don't want to go. The game will be a big hassle. Parking will be impossible—there'll be too many people. We're not going."

When Luke thought about it, he realized that his father wasn't going much of anywhere these days. He mostly stayed around the house and almost always looked tired. One night Luke woke up late, startled by a noise from down the hall. He got up to go to the bathroom and noticed a light on in the living room. He peeked in and saw his dad sitting there with his head in his hands. Luke didn't like seeing him like that, and he walked into the room and said softly, "Dad?" His father looked up quickly and Luke saw in the light of the lamp that his face looked awful. He looked much older, exhausted, and sad.

"Dad? Is everything OK?"

"It's OK, Luke," his father said. He shook his head.

Luke went over and sat down on the couch next to him. "What's wrong?"

"Nothing. I just had a bad dream, that's all. Shook me up a little bit. But it's all right. It was just a dream."

Luke put his arm around his father the way his father had for him when he was sad, and they sat like that for a few minutes. The next morning, Luke woke up to find himself stretched out on the couch with a blanket over him. His dad was still sitting there, looking out the window.

His father seemed to get quieter as the days went by, except for when he got angry. If Luke woke up during the night, he often found him on the couch, watching the Military Channel or staring off into space. Luke's parents seemed to fight a lot. They didn't like to argue in front of the kids, but Luke always knew they were upset because they would go quiet when he walked into the room and wouldn't look at each other.

Luke asked his mom about it once and she said she thought his dad was having trouble with some of the things he had seen in Iraq. "What kind of things?" Luke asked.

"Soldiers see a lot of hard things when they're at war," his mom explained. "Sometimes they see people get hurt and they want to help them or protect them and they can't. It isn't always easy to know how to deal with those things. Besides," she added, "your father was gone for over a year. You and Beth both grew up and changed a lot while he was gone. He loves you so much, it makes him sad to feel like he missed that time with you."

She paused, then went on. "You just wait. Your dad is working through some things. But he'll be going back to work soon, and he won't have as much time to think. He'll be fine then. You'll see."

Luke's dad went back to work a few days later, putting his uniform back on and heading off to the base each morning. At first, as Luke's mother had predicted, he did seem to cheer up. He came home one day laughing about a story he had shared with one of his buddies, and for the first time since he got back, he looked like the dad that Luke remembered.

But that didn't last long. Driving back from the base each day seemed to make him crazy. Day after day he came home furious with some driver on the highway who had been going too fast. Unlike the calm, funny father Luke remembered, now when he got mad, his father seemed to stay mad for a long time.

All through dinner he would continue ranting about other drivers on the highway, still angry that their driving was so reckless. He seemed unable to calm back down. Luke's dad had always had a beer with dinner, but now he was having another in front of the TV after the dishes were done, and sometimes when Luke woke up in the night he found him there with the TV still on, sleeping on the couch with a couple of bottles on the table beside him. Luke hid them in the trash so his mom wouldn't see. She hated it when his father drank.

But the turning point came one night a few weeks later. Luke woke to the sound of Beth crying, and it seemed to be coming from his parents' room. He walked in there groggily and found his mother holding Beth on her lap, rocking gently.

On the other side of the room, his father was pacing back and forth across the carpet. His face was sweaty and he was very pale. His mother said nothing, but her mouth was set the way it got when she had made up her mind about something. "What happened?" Luke asked. His father looked up at him then walked out of the room.

Luke's mother put her hand on Beth's hair and whispered, "Shhhhhh" in her ear. She turned to Luke and said, "Your father had another one of his dreams about the war. He has them sometimes and wakes up shouting or waving around with his hands. But Beth was sleeping in the bed with us, and he woke up shaking her, thinking that she was someone trying to hurt him in his dream. She's fine, but it scared her, and your dad's upset that he might have hurt her."

The next morning, Luke's parents drove over to the Behavioral Health Clinic on base. There they saw a doctor and told her what had been going on with Luke's dad at home: the dreams, the trouble sleeping, the irritability and inability to calm down. The doctor said that these were common signs of post-traumatic stress disorder, PTSD for short, which is an illness that people who have experienced very stressful or upsetting events sometimes develop, including soldiers who have served in a war zone like Iraq.

The doctor told Luke's parents that while PTSD can be difficult for a soldier and his or her family, there are very good treatments available. She said that Luke's dad would get better once he got some help. They made an appointment for him to see a psychologist, someone who helps people learn to deal with their feelings.

The next few weeks were tough, but there were hopeful signs. The whole family had been frightened by what had happened that night in Luke's parents' room, so Luke's dad started sleeping on the couch, just in case he had one of his dreams. He completely stopped drinking, even his beer with dinner, because the doctor said that alcohol can interfere with sleeping and worsen other symptoms. He still got irritable when driving, and with Beth and Luke when they were loud, but since the doctor had told him that his quick temper was a sign of PTSD, he made a special effort to calm himself down before yelling or getting too mad.

After Luke's father began seeing the psychologist, he went into Luke's room one night and tried to explain what was going on. "Luke," he said, "I want you to understand what is happening with me, because I'm really happy with the psychologist and I feel like the treatment is working. I want you to know that it's all going to be all right."

"So what's wrong with you?" Luke asked. He knew that he didn't sound very respectful, but he was frustrated by all that had been going on and didn't really care.

His dad was very big on respect, but he didn't get mad that Luke spoke so directly. Instead he said, "Son, war is a terrible thing. Sometimes I think it's a necessary thing, which is why I became a soldier. But it's a terrible thing and causes a lot of pain for everybody involved. I knew when I got back that I was going to have trouble with some of the things that happened over there."

"So why didn't you do something about it then?" Luke asked.

His father paused for a long time before replying. "There were a couple of reasons. Because I was hoping it would take care of itself. Because I was so happy to be home with you all that I didn't want to focus on anything negative. And because I was afraid that you all might think less of me for admitting that I was having problems. Sometimes it takes a lot of courage to admit that you're having a hard time, and I wasn't sure I had any courage left. But when I saw that my problems were starting to affect my family, that was it. That's not allowed. And I'm really glad that I got some help."

Luke thought about this, then said, "But I still don't get it. Why did you come back so different?"

His father sighed. "When I was over in Iraq, I saw how war can hurt people. Many people die in combat and even more people are injured. A lot of the time I was over there I was really angry and worried and sometimes really scared. Soldiers and marines and other guys like me don't like to talk about being scared, but we do—we get scared like anybody else."

Luke nodded.

"When you live like that for a long time," his dad continued, "your mind and your body get used to it and you start to react to the world around you differently. You get used to reacting very quickly and instinctively because you have to just to survive. But then when you come home, it's hard to turn that back off. That's why I've been so on edge lately. I'm really sorry if I've been hard on you and your sister—you two are the most important people in the world to me—but now that I can understand why I am this way, the psychologist at the clinic is helping me learn how to control it better."

"What about the dreams?" Luke said. "Why do you get like that in your sleep?"

"Well, sometimes the things I saw over in Iraq come back to me when I'm sleeping. But I've been talking to the psychologist about that, too, and it seems like talking to him about those things has been easing up the dreams. The psychologist says that he doesn't think I will have dreams like that after we finish the treatment. I may still have bad dreams, but they won't be nearly as intense, and I won't be at risk of lashing out at you kids or your mom, which is my biggest concern."

Luke was quiet for a while. His dad sat there patiently, waiting for him to speak. Finally Luke said, "So does this mean you're not going to be so angry all the time?"

"I hope so, Luke. I'm working on it."

"And maybe you'll leave the house sometimes, besides for work?"

His dad snorted, then smiled. "Yeah, that too."

"OK." Luke shrugged. His dad reached out, pulled Luke close for a hug, and said, "I love you, Buddy." Then he got up and left Luke to his homework.

After their talk, things continued much as they had since his father got back from Iraq, but with small shifts that made all the difference. Luke noticed that his dad wasn't complaining so much during dinner and once in a while cracked a joke or two. He was more patient with Luke and his sister, and when they did get in trouble, he didn't yell about it or stomp out of the room. Luke stopped finding his father in the living room in the middle of the night and eventually stopped waking up to nighttime noises all together. He no longer walked into the kitchen and found his parents silent, avoiding each other's eyes. Instead, after his father's many months away, he again got used to seeing his father helping his mom with dinner, talking and sharing stories about work or other daily things.

And one day Luke came home after school to find an envelope with his name on it on the kitchen table. He opened it up to find four tickets to that Friday's Spurs game and a note from his dad. It read simply, "Think Jimmy and his dad might want to go?"

14

Tenzin's Dream

Sara Lewis

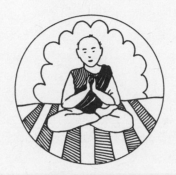

In "Tenzin's Dream," a teenage Tibetan refugee describes how letting go of negative emotions helped her cope with political violence back in Tibet. Many Tibetans have experienced persecution and sometimes torture since the Chinese began occupying their land. Tibetans began escaping to Nepal and northern India in the 1950s, and in doing so they faced an arduous journey. Despite working at a mobile phone shop together for many months, Tenzin had never shared her history as a former political prisoner with her Indian friend, Lakshmi. Through asking questions about her experience, Lakshmi learns that Tenzin has coped with these difficult experiences not through talking and sharing with others but by creating space and flexibility in her mind through Buddhist practices. It is customary in Tibetan Buddhism to deal with negative emotion in this way, through recognizing them and focusing on compassion. This story illustrates the important link between mind training and negative emotion and demonstrates the powerful role that the mind can have in coping with difficult situations.

Lakshmi shivered as she took another sip of chai. "I'm bored," she said.

"You're always bored," teased Tenzin. "Should we have more chai?"

Lakshmi and Tenzin sat huddled together sipping cups of chai tea. Lakshmi wore a *salwaar kameez*, and Tenzin wore jeans and a hooded sweat shirt. Both girls had several woolen blankets wrapped tightly around them to block the icy winds streaming into the windows of their shop.

Perched on a hill of their small town located in the foothills of the Himalayas, large snow-capped mountains framed their view. A few months ago, Tenzin, a nineteen-year-old Tibetan refugee, started working at the small mobile phone shop owned by Lakshmi's father. Lakshmi's father never intended to hire staff outside his family, but with so many Tibetans around town, he needed someone who could communicate with those who did not speak Hindi or English. Lakshmi often worked at the shop as she studied for her college entrance exam. She hoped to go to nursing school somewhere warm in the south of India, but her parents worried she would not be safe so far away—three whole days of travel by train.

To pass the time at work, Lakshmi and Tenzin often would sit side by side, each doing their studies. Other times they would spend the entire day talking. Today was too cold to sit still. Lakshmi jumped up and began bouncing up and down. "It's freezing today," she complained as she tried to warm her toes.

Tenzin smiled, watching her friend. She looked completely silly, wrapped in a blanket, her *dupatta* scarf flapping underneath as she bounced around the room to keep warm. After a few minutes, Lakshmi flopped down beside Tenzin.

"Should we go on Facebook?" asked Lakshmi. She had begged her brother earlier in the day to leave his laptop at the shop. The girls looked through photos taken by a boy who was an old schoolmate of Lakshmi. They giggled and cringed at a picture of him trying to ride a motorcycle.

Their attention was suddenly diverted from Facebook as a muffled noise outside their window became louder. The window panes were covered in plastic hastily taped to the walls to keep out the frigid February air, so they found a loose corner in the plastic to peer through and saw a line of Tibetans coming down the street. Many were monks and nuns dressed in maroon and saffron robes with layered sweaters. A number of laypeople joined them; both young and old marched together.

"*Bod Gyalo*! Victory to Tibet!" one teenage boy screamed, holding up a photo of a woman who had recently committed suicide by setting herself on fire back in Tibet. She joined dozens of others who have self-immolated as a form protest. It was unclear for whom the boy was displaying the photo, but Tenzin guessed that his anger came from the violence that the Chinese had inflicted on the Tibetan people in order to occupy their land and destroy their culture. Many Tibetans were angry. But most of the crowd was more subdued. Some were holding candles, and many collectively recited Buddhist mantras of peace.

Tenzin gazed out the window at the march and sighed deeply. These marches were becoming more common, and she worried that things would not get better.

Tenzin came to India from Tibet when she was eighteen years old in order to get an education. She didn't consider herself to be someone very interested in politics. Mostly she was interested in her studies and music. She had grown up in a small farming village in eastern Tibet and at age sixteen had lost her mother in a bus accident.

Although she had attended a few years of primary school at a Chinese-run schoolhouse, Tenzin generally stayed at home to help her family with the farm and to look after their small herd of yaks and sheep. After her mother died, she told her father she wanted to go to India to attend school. She spoke little Chinese, and most schools were not allowed to teach in the Tibetan language. Her uncle had taught her the Tibetan alphabet, but she was ashamed she could barely read and write her native language. It was her dream to study Tibetan literature and poetry.

Sometimes people left books at the monastery and her uncle would save them for Tenzin. Over the years she had acquired an impressive collection of books she proudly displayed on a small shelf above her bed in Tibet. She meticulously cleaned the dust off the shelf every week, running her fingers along the golden Tibetan lettering on the binding of the book covers.

Tenzin's father didn't want her to leave. He feared she would be arrested and maybe even put in prison, as many Tibetans who tried to escape China were. When Tenzin's uncle, a monk at their local monastery, decided to leave, her father reluctantly allowed her to join the small group of Tibetans planning their journey through Nepal and into India. She did not know very much about the political situation, but she wanted more than anything to go to school.

The noises from the march reminded Tenzin of the loud, sharp voices of the female prison guards in Lhasa. She quickly picked up her *mala* (prayer beads) and silently recited the mantra of Tara, looking at the floor.

"What's up?" asked Lakshmi, taking Tenzin back to the present.

"Oh, nothing," said Tenzin. She put down her mala and picked up her English homework. "I have two classes today," she said with a look of determination. Tenzin attended two or three hours of English class every day at a local nonprofit organization, before and after work at the shop. They didn't have a regular teacher, but sometimes young foreign travelers volunteered their time by facilitating English conversation classes.

"Your English is so good, Tenzin," said Lakshmi approvingly with a slight wobble of her head from side to side, showing respect. "It is impressive you learned so much English in a year, without even attending a proper school!"

Tenzin blushed and looked down at her notebook. She thought back to her elation at finally making it to India and her devastation when she learned she was too old to attend the Tibetan schools. She was given a small stipend by the Tibetan government-in-exile and offered a place in a trade school where she could learn to cook. But the school was twelve hours away and Tenzin wanted to stay close to her uncle, who had been taken in by a nearby monastery. Besides, she was not ready to give up on her dream of learning to read all those books she had left behind in Tibet. But she also needed to work, and her neighbors told her she would need to concentrate on learning English if she was going to survive in India. Life in exile was not as she had imagined it.

Almost as if she was reading Tenzin's mind, Lakshmi said, "You don't talk much about your homeland. You must miss your father."

"It does not help to talk of such things," said Tenzin matter-of-factly. "We just have to keep going and not become too sad. One day I will return when things are better there."

Lakshmi sensed that Tenzin had had a difficult past. Although they mostly spent their time giggling over chai and taking photos on their mobile phones, sometimes a dark and heavy look would fall across Tenzin's ruddy, windswept face. Lakshmi wanted to ask Tenzin about her journey to India. After all, she often told Tenzin stories about growing up in India. The girls would laugh when Lakshmi's brother did funny impersonations of their many aunts and uncles, and Tenzin knew all the details of Lakshmi's childhood.

But Tenzin didn't talk about herself. She never complained about being homesick. In fact, she never seemed to complain about anything. Although Lakshmi hoped to go on to nursing school down south, she also felt a pang of sadness in her heart when she imagined being away from her parents and older brothers. Lakshmi knew that Tenzin also had older brothers, but she rarely mentioned them. Sometimes she would look at a small collection of old photos she kept in her bag.

Both Indians and Tibetans live together in this small town, but mostly Indians associated with other Indians and Tibetans with other Tibetans. When Tenzin started working at the shop, the girls were cordial to each other but a little shy. In just a matter of weeks, however, they quickly bonded, becoming fast friends. Lakshmi did not know very much about the Tibetan and Chinese political situation. But like most of her Indian friends and relatives, they felt proud to live close to the Dalai Lama, despite the underlying tension between locals and the growing Tibetan population.

Lakshmi wanted to show her support for Tenzin. As the group of protesters passed down the street, Lakshmi said rather awkwardly, "It is not right, how so many people are arrested in Tibet."

The girls sat in silence.

Unsure of what to say next, Lakshmi asked, "Do you know anyone who went to prison?"

Tenzin shifted nervously in her seat. "Yes, of course," she said.

"Many people in my county were arrested after the monks at our local monastery didn't allow Chinese police to inspect the grounds."

"That's awful," said Lakshmi. "Here in India, the police wouldn't dare to upset our Hindu gods, marching into a temple."

Suddenly Tenzin began to cry. Usually it was Lakshmi who displayed all the emotion.

"I was in a prison," said Tenzin quietly. At that moment a group of monks came into the shop to recharge their mobile-phone balances.

Lakshmi stood in silence while Tenzin helped each monk recharge his balance in the same small increment: fifty rupees, or about one U.S. dollar. After the monks left, the girls again sat in silence. Tenzin wondered why she had mentioned prison to Lakshmi. This was not something she often talked about, even with other Tibetans who also had been in prison.

Finally Lakshmi spoke. "Tenzin, we are friends. It's not good to hold in your feelings. I tell my mother and my cousins everything, which always makes me feel better. It's good to share things with others."

Tenzin didn't want to hide anything from Lakshmi, but she worried that speaking very openly about her imprisonment would stir up too many negative emotions. She tightened the wool blanket she had wrapped around her waist. The Tibetan grandmothers around town often scolded the young women for not properly keeping their kidneys warm. "You will become sick!" her elderly neighbor told her nearly every morning. She secretly enjoyed these scoldings, which made her feel cared for.

Tenzin still missed her mother. But she often held in her tears. It will not help, it will not bring her back, she would tell herself. Instead she would offer some butter lamps at a nearby nunnery or circumambulate around the main temple, a Tibetan Buddhist practice that involves walking clockwise around a holy structure or sacred place. Many believe that through showing respect to these places of power, they will purify negative karma and gain merit, or good karma.

Doing these practices, Tenzin offered the merit or good karma she generated to her mother, praying that she took a good rebirth. This always made Tenzin feel better. It calmed her mind and she felt she was doing something positive to help. Her parents taught her that sitting around with negative emotions, such as sadness and anger, was only harmful. It never helped the situation, and these feelings could even make you sick. Just like cold and severe weather can disrupt the balance in the body, negative feelings could affect one's mind.

Her uncle always reminded her to keep her mind calm and stable. "No matter what," he would say, "if you can keep your mind calm—not getting too upset or too elated—this is very healthy. In life we are faced with a mix of good times and bad times. You have to train your mind to remain calm in the face of anything. This also ensures you don't create more and more bad karma. When something happens, just accept that you are purifying your karma and try not to react too strongly. It won't help the situation and will only create more suffering."

These words echoed in Tenzin's mind as she considered what Lakshmi had said.

"It wasn't so bad," Tenzin shared. "Many Tibetans are arrested when they try to cross the border. I only had to stay for a few months. Other people are kept in prison for years and beaten severely. It wasn't so bad for me."

"That is really terrible that you were arrested, Tenzin," said Lakshmi. "I never knew. And I'm just confused because you don't really seem interested in the political protests here. I never imagined that something like that happened to you."

"It's all right. It's over now. And now I am moving forward in my life. This is just my karma," Tenzin replied.

Tenzin's response made Lakshmi feel uncomfortable. She did not understand how Tenzin could act as if being a former political prisoner was no big deal. Lakshmi sat silently for a few minutes, looking out the window at the monks and nuns marching in the street. Their neatly pressed maroon-and-saffron robes looked elegant in stark contrast to the dusty Indian streets lined with potato chip wrappers, plastic bottles, and discarded paper.

A group of young men in their early twenties came into the shop, laughing loudly with their arms around one another. "Want a Snickers bar?" one said to Tenzin and Lakshmi.

"No, thank you," said both girls in unison. They looked at each other and smiled. The shift in energy was a welcome respite from the previous moments of heavy emotion. One of the young men began playing a recent Bollywood hit on his phone. The group cheered, and one mimicked some dance moves while singing to Lakshmi. Lakshmi glanced over at Tenzin, rolling her eyes as if to say *give me a break*. After looking at the latest model of iPhone, the group left the shop.

"Listen," said Lakshmi, "you can still hear them carrying on, down the street!" Tenzin smiled and the girls chatted about the cold weather for the remainder of the day—neither wanting to mention what Tenzin had shared. Around six o'clock they began closing the shop. Lakshmi counted the money and Tenzin straightened the merchandise and swept the floor.

"Are you going to English class now?" asked Lakshmi.

Tenzin paused for a moment. "Actually, I might go down to the temple. Would you like to join me?"

Despite their growing friendship at work, Tenzin and Lakshmi did not spend time together outside the shop. After work Lakshmi would walk to the bus to head home, and Tenzin would go down the footpath to the Tibetan area of town. But Lakshmi appreciated the invitation and was eager to try to repair the awkwardness of the day's events.

"Yes, I'd love to," Lakshmi replied. The girls walked, hand in hand, down the road to the large Buddhist temple where many Tibetan community members gathered for evening prayers. Some older Tibetans were clustered together on long wooden planks, doing hundreds of prostrations in succession to purify negative karma. Holding their hands in prayer position, they gestured to their head, throat, and heart, symbolizing the purification of body, speech, and mind. Using bits of cloth to help ease them downward, they slowly slid until their foreheads touched the ground.

"It's very good for your body. The prostrations," said Tenzin, looking over at the older people. The girls joined the groups of Tibetans making *kora*, or circumambulating the temple. Many fingered their prayer beads, reciting streams of mantras under their breath. Some were spinning prayer wheels, sending out sacred mantras into the wind. Tenzin and Lakshmi walked in silence. But it was not the same awkward silence they had experienced in the shop earlier that day. It was calm and peaceful.

Lakshmi hadn't spent much time within the walls of the Tibetan monastery. Many tourists came inside every day, taking photographs and strolling about. But as an Indian resident, she mostly stayed in her own neighborhood. Plus, she never knew exactly what to do at the Buddhist temple, which was different from the Hindu temple she visited with her family. But she felt at ease walking alongside Tenzin, who silently recited mantras next to her.

"What are these candles, exactly?" asked Lakshmi, gesturing to a large table of flickering lights, homemade from melted butter.

"Those are butter lamps. We offer them and wish for the health and well-being of all living, spiritual beings. Or sometimes we light them for specific people if they are sick or have recently died."

"I could stand by these lights forever. They're beautiful." The hundreds of neatly placed butter lamps flickered and sparked as the butter slowly melted away the cloth wicks. Without speaking, the girls, seemingly in unison, walked away from the butter lamps to rejoin the crowd doing their evening practices. Some people were chatting with relatives and neighbors. Others looked deep in prayer. The crowd meandered around the inner part of the temple. Some young people gently skirted around an old man hunched over a walking stick, shuffling along the path. Tenzin and Lakshmi continued circumambulating the temple for a while longer before deciding to go and have some tea.

"Lakshmi, I have never seen you so quiet," joked Tenzin. "Did you enjoy the temple?"

Lakshmi smiled back at Tenzin. "Yes! I feel very calm, both in my body and my mind. It's a little strange. I just feel very open."

"As Buddhists, we come here to make offerings and do practices to purify our negative karma. And this is important. But it really helps me calm my mind. Just as you're saying. That open and calm feeling."

"Yes," said Lakshmi. "I can see how this would help." The girls sipped their tea and watched the sea of monks, nuns, and laypeople walking down the hill to the monastery. "You know," continued Lakshmi, "about today . . ." she said, trailing off.

"It's OK," replied Tenzin. "It's not that I am trying to hide anything from you."

Lakshmi listened to Tenzin with great interest. "I understand that. But if you just hold it all inside and keep it to yourself, doesn't that just make it worse?"

"I actually asked my uncle that same question when we were back in Tibet. After my mother died, I cried and cried. I would wail loudly at night for my mother. I was sixteen years old, but I felt like a small child. My relatives felt very sorry for me and tried to help me." Tenzin paused and sipped her tea. "But then," she continued, "I had a talk with my uncle that really helped me. My uncle is a very wise man who has studied many years to become a monk and knows a great deal about Tibetan practice."

"What did he say?" asked Lakshmi.

"My uncle told me that it is only natural to be sad. My mother showed me great love and kindness, and everyone feels this way when they lose their mother. He sat with me and asked me to visualize all the other people on the planet who right then, at that very moment, had lost their mother and were feeling just like me. This was not difficult to do. Actually it had not even occurred to me that also my brothers had lost their mother. And my father, his wife. I was so trapped in my own suffering that I didn't even realize I wasn't the only one feeling this way. And then I thought about some friends who had also lost a parent. I knew many others felt this way. They, too, lost their precious mother. I sat there with my uncle for a long time. I kept thinking and expanding my mind further. I realized that every person eventually loses their mother. Even my own mother lost her mother. I said to my uncle, 'Why do I feel better?' My mind for the first time since she has been gone is feeling more calm.'"

"And then?" asked Lakshmi, nodding with interest.

"He explained that as we get older and become more wise and

mature, we have to learn how to cope with problems like losing our parents and other difficult experiences. Young children don't yet understand how to cope very well. We have to learn to be resilient, to have strength to carry on in spite of challenges in life. Resilience comes through making the mind more spacious and flexible. As we say in Tibetan, *sems pa chen po*, a 'broad and vast mind.'"

Lakshmi listened intently. "I'm not sure I understand, exactly."

Tenzin sat for a few moments in silence. Finally she said, "When you are right in the middle of a problem and overwhelmed by emotion, it is like a tidal wave. You are completely caught and you cannot see beyond what you are feeling. The mind becomes very narrow and unstable. A vast and spacious mind provides room to accommodate instability. Misfortune and disappointment is only natural. We have to be realistic and not be surprised when we encounter difficulty. We know from the Buddhist teachings that all feelings and emotions are impermanent; they do not last."

Tenzin smiled at her friend and continued. "Those with spacious minds can see beyond what is happening in the moment. They realize that these feelings will not last. When I was crying for my mother, I couldn't see beyond the emotion. It seemed it would last forever and never end. My uncle explained that we cling to emotions and make them very solid—even if they are negative. And this is harmful to both the mind and body."

Tenzin paused to make sure her friend was following her. When Lakshmi nodded, she went on. "When I thought of all the others in the same situation as me, my sadness didn't disappear. But it brought more space into my mind, meaning that I was able to feel compassion for all the others also grieving for their mother. And where there is compassion, there is always more space. I remained sad for a very long time. And I am still sad. But with time I can see that my sadness is not fixed and solid."

"So, you're able to bring more space into your mind by focusing on others?" asked Lakshmi.

"Yes," Tenzin said. "When we're doing these practices on behalf of others, we turn the attention away from ourselves. We focus on doing something positive and bringing peace into the world for all beings. We recognize that actually we're all trapped in *samsara*, the cycle of rebirth, which traps those who have not yet become enlightened. Really, we are all in the same situation. There are many practices and Buddhist teachings that help us to think in this way. There are teachings called *lojong*, or 'mind training,' which help us to broaden our thinking in difficult situations. When I was arrested and put in prison there was one very humble nun there with me who taught me some lojong. She explained that the idea is to completely reverse our habitual thinking. Normally, we focus on ourselves. But this only creates more and more suffering. It doesn't actually help us. But by wishing for others to be happy, we become much more patient and calm. It doesn't mean we do not feel any emotion. But we are better able to let emotions go. Now whenever I start to think about the difficulties I faced in prison, I just think, It's over now. This was your karma. You have purified it and now it is over. It does not help me to hold on to the suffering from the past."

"I understand now why you were reluctant to talk about your experience."

"I guess this is my habit now, to try to let go. Those who are very humble and skillful will think, The more peaceful and calm my mind, the more I am able to help others. Sometimes I do get very upset when I think about my time in prison. When this happens I try to have compassion for myself. I also try to build compassion for others around the world who are in prison. I even think that we could feel compassion for the prison guards. They are probably good people. But they are creating very negative karma and they are really the ones who will suffer in the long run, when they are reborn. I try to generate compassion for the entire situation. This does not completely make my feelings go away. But widening my perspective helps me to cope."

Lakshmi nodded and felt that she had learned something. Not just about Tenzin but about a new way of approaching problems. Tenzin and Lakshmi had long finished their tea. But both wanted to sit just a little while longer.

Sangath
Kathy Wollner

Sangath is an organization committed to improving health for people of all ages. In India, where Sangath operates, there is a very large gap between the number of people who need mental health care and the people available to deliver it, such as psychiatrists, psychologists, and other counselors. Sangath seeks to close this gap and provide more people with mental health care that can greatly improve their quality of life.

Sangath started its work in 1996 in Goa, India, with a child development clinic. This was an interdisciplinary clinic, which means it included health providers from different backgrounds all in one place. Sangath believes that a mix of social, psychological, and medical interventions is needed for community health. Now Sangath is one of the most influential organizations in India and has become an example for other countries around the world, including high-income nations like the United States.

Unfortunately, most of India lacks affordable health services. Sangath uses resources—especially human resources—already present in communities. The organization trains people without prior training in mental health care and supervises them so they can serve their own communities. Sangath's activities include the following:

- Teaching health counselors how to provide counseling for people with mental illness
- Bringing health counselors into schools
- Integrating learning resource rooms and remedial education in schools to make schools more accessible to young people with learning disabilities

161

- Training community outreach workers to promote the mental health of people living with HIV and their caregivers

Sangath has a number of exciting programs. One focuses on implementing a counseling program for depression and harmful alcohol drinking at primary health centers. Another teaches parents how to provide the best support possible for their children with autism. Sangath also conducts research on mental health care in India, which is used to improve their mental health treatment services. The researchers at Sangath recently completed research studies evaluating how lay counselors can be used to identify and treat common mental disorders through community-based rehabilitation. This model places care and treatment in the community rather than at a hospital, where mental health care has traditionally been carried out. Sangath's studies have addressed a wide spectrum of mental disorders, from depression to schizophrenia. This research is important because it lets Sangath know if the model it uses to improve mental health care is working.

DISCUSSION QUESTIONS

- What do you learn about mental health and well-being in your school?
- Do you have someone you can turn to, such as a health counselor, at school? If not, what would having a health counselor change about your school environment?
- Where do people with mental illness get care and treatment in your community? Is there a treatment gap, meaning there are more people who need treatment than who have access to treatment?
- Find an organization working to improve care for people with mental illness and/or people with disabilities in your community. What methods does this organization use to improve care? How are they different from or similar to Sangath's methods?

- Some organizations are skeptical about the idea of training lay-people to deliver mental health care. Why do you think this is? What arguments would you use to convince them it is possible?

This section's information has been adapted from Sangath's website. To learn more about Sangath, visit www.sangath.org.

Section IV

Violence

Violence has always been part of human society. It can be interpersonal violence, such as gun violence between people, or structural violence, meaning that the social conditions in which someone lives can cause harm. The complexity of violence in people's lives can be difficult to measure and see. But understanding how violence can influence a person's mental and physical health is a fundamental part of community health.

Interpersonal violence, which is defined as a violent act inflicted by one person or party on another, is an incredibly important issue for community health. The impact of such violence on a person's mental health was demonstrated in "A Homecoming," where observing extreme forms of interpersonal violence during wartime caused Luke's dad to develop PTSD. Interpersonal violence describes many kinds of violence, some obvious and others subtle. Emotional, physical, and sexual abuse can all cause physical and emotional pain. Emotional abuse includes being bullied or put down by others, sexual abuse includes rape or molestation, and physical abuse includes things like being hit or kicked by another person. Gun violence, another form of interpersonal violence, often leads to serious injury and even death. Being a witness to abuse can be traumatic as well.

But violence is not always visible. A common term used to describe this often-invisible harm is *structural violence*. Structural violence means that social structures outside of individuals' control, such as poverty and unemployment, prevent them from meeting basic needs, such as eating healthy foods and finding sustainable housing. This means that disease may not result from the choices one makes but from larger problems such as poverty and poor working conditions. For example, if a family lives near a river and waste from a factory contaminates the water upstream, the family's water supply may be unsafe. That family's sickness, then, results from the inability to find a cleaner water source, a problem caused by the factory not following regulations for waste disposal. Another example is HIV and AIDS. Many of those affected by HIV and AIDS are children. Some children are born with the disease and must live with the virus their whole lives, while others, who are not HIV positive, are nonetheless affected by the disease because they lose a parent or sibling. In this case, their suffering is a result of association with the virus.

In many cases, both visible and less visible violence can cause poor health many years after the violence takes place. This section is very much related to the previous section on mental health because violence can affect people's mental health and ability to cope with everyday life. While it is clear how infections or tumors can cause disease, the stress caused by experiences, such as Luke's father's military combat, can be more difficult to measure and understand. In some cases, even witnessing violence can cause severe mental distress. However, anxiety or depression can also result from the stress of living in poverty. This may endure for many years.

Other types of violence, such as bullying and discrimination, can also affect people's health and well-being. By treating people who are different from you badly, you can have a negative impact on their health. Accepting people for who they are by showing compassion and understanding promotes healthy communities. Violence from fists, knives, or guns can have more direct effects on a person's health. People may come away from fights with bruises and broken bones, or more serious injuries like knife or gunshot wounds, which can cause serious injury or even death. Unfortunately, homicide is the third leading cause of death among young people age ten to twenty-four.* These deaths often cause great stress on families and can affect entire communities. Those who do survive violence often suffer health problems from their injuries for years to come.

This section describes the ways in which violence can influence people's physical and mental health. In "Paris of the West," Juliana

---

* Centers for Disease Control, 2010, http://www.cdc.gov/violenceprevention/youthviolence/stats_at-a_glance/lcd_10-24.html/.

experiences sexual violence at five years of age, resulting in a lifelong impact on her mental health. "We All Fight" demonstrates how rural poverty on the Blackfeet Reservation in Montana can have an impact on people's lives, contributing to risk taking and injury. Risk taking also plays a role in "Nelson's Soweto," a story that highlights the effect of gun violence in people's lives through Nelson and his friends' experiences in urban South Africa. "The Grove" demonstrates how the conditions that people are born into are often unequal and can shape health outcomes.

As you read through this section, consider the following questions:

- How might interpersonal violence influence someone's health? For example, how might physical injury as a result of gun violence or rape affect a person's physical or mental health?

- Have you or someone you know ever experienced or witnessed gun violence? How did you or your friend cope with it?

- Is bullying violence? Is discrimination violence? How can bullying and discrimination affect people's health? What can you do to work against bullying or discrimination in your school or community?

15
Paris of the West

Ember Keighley

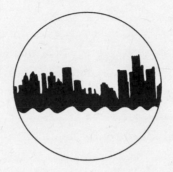

"Paris of the West" introduces how child sexual abuse can have a negative impact on a person's life. First abused when she was five, Juliana held this secret close to her until she was a teenager. She carried the burden of this secret through her childhood and well into her teens, until a teacher encouraged her to speak with someone. Contemplating suicide and suffering from severe depression, Juliana visits a small free clinic and meets a doctor who makes her feel comfortable and with whom she shares her story. This story underscores the importance of recognizing the role of abuse in young people's lives and how debilitating holding on to such a memory can be. Nearly one in five women in the United States report being sexually abused during their lifetime. This type of severe interpersonal violence requires social and often medical support. Many people feel shame and fear related to the violence they experienced, and sharing one's story with a close friend or a counselor can make a big difference.

Detroit was once called the Paris of the West. You can see it every once in a while. It is in the ornate gilding of the downtown buildings, with their meticulously carved designs and towering ceilings. They look so grand that you expect to see people dressed in their finest gowns around every corner. But there is no one. Those elegant buildings are empty in the middle of the day. It is in the beautiful stone fountains without water. It is in the train station, which once served as the great welcoming center to people from all over the world but now lies underneath an overpass. Its glorious arching doorways and soaring windows beckon only pigeons on their travels. Most days you can walk across the street without looking because there are no cars. At night, the tall elegant skyscrapers reveal their hidden secret: there is no one there to turn their lights on. The city is dark.

Detroit was once hopeful and vibrant. It boasted the best and newest cars. It was host to great artists from all over the world. Then the jobs disappeared with the auto industry, and the race riots sent those white folks who had stayed running to the suburbs, taking their business and jobs with them. Now the Paris of the West stands mostly empty and alone, the bare foundation of what it used to be.

But to Juliana, Detroit was home. She could see herself reflected in the city she grew up in. As she sat in the now-cold bathtub shivering, she imagined a time when she too felt complete, whole. It was hard to imagine. She was now as empty inside as those skyscrapers. Like those old buildings, she wished there was someone to turn her lights on and care for her. She could not remember what it was like not to feel empty and hollow. All of these thoughts danced through her head as her lips touched the water. Juliana so frequently doubted why she was alive. Was there any hope? Could she ever feel normal again? Her baths often started this way.

Just after slipping into the tub, taking a breath, and sinking into the water until her lips touched the surface, a flood of guilt always overwhelmed her. Erin was only two. Who would raise her daughter without her? She surrendered and breathed again at the thought of Erin's tiny cornrows with pink and purple barrettes at the ends.

"Juliana!" she heard her mother yell from downstairs. Reluctantly, she lifted herself out of tub and picked her towel up from its heap on the floor. As she hurried to dry her shivering body, she caught her reflection in the mirror. Juliana never liked the image looking back at her.

Her arms were thin and frail, her hair was messy with her braids falling out, her face was long, her eyes looked tired, and her cheek was scarred. She looked away as quickly as she had looked and slipped on the same clothes from the pile on the floor. Then she ran downstairs before her mom became more irritated.

"What have you been doing? You leave me here alone to watch *your* daughter while you waste time doing nothing. At least be useful for something and go get dinner. And you had better be finishing your homework. I am sick of having to talk to teachers about you." Her mother held out a crumpled bill and gestured toward the door with one hand while the other held a cigarette with long ashes waiting to fall on the table.

As Juliana reached for the bill, her mother blew the smoke in her face. Juliana took the bill without looking at her mother, slipped on her old shoes, and hurried out the door. "Barney's coming over," she heard her mother say as she slammed the door and ran down the crumbling cement steps without locking it. She would have to hear about that later, but she didn't care. Being yelled at was inevitable, and she resented everything about her mom's boyfriend.

Juliana opened the door to the convenience store with the neon ATM sign. She glanced down at the bill in her hands, a ten. That was never enough. It was the end of the month and that would have to last them the next two days. Her mother must have bought Barney beer again, she thought. She headed to the aisle with dinner food and grabbed two boxes of macaroni and cheese, Erin's favorite, and one loaf of bread. She quickly added up the prices in her head, not enough for peanut butter, she thought, and grabbed one more box of macaroni and cheese instead. She would be hungry tomorrow. There were no grocery stores in Detroit.

Juliana had seen the pictures on TV of aisles full of fruits and vegetables. She wondered how people could afford those. The vegetables in the free school lunches never appealed to her. They always looked a little old and slimy, and they didn't make her feel full anyway. As far as she was concerned, it seemed like a waste to get those when you could put something on your tray that would fill you. She had never seen a store like those ones on TV. Everyone she knew ate food from the convenience stores. It was just the way things were in Detroit. Maybe in the suburbs, where the wealthy people lived, there were stores like that.

Barney looked her up and down when she walked in the door with the plastic bag of groceries in her hand. She rushed to close the door while his eyes paused at her breasts and the button of her jeans. He winked at her when his eyes reached her face. Her stomach churned. She rushed into the kitchen and away from Barney's gaze as fast as she could, but still she couldn't halt the overwhelming memories.

Juliana dreaded the days when Barney was over. They made the hollow emptiness that always lurched in her soul flood with guilt. They made her mind flash back to the images she fought so hard to keep away. How could that first man have touched her when she was so young? She had not been that many years older than Erin when it first happened. She had had no way to defend herself or any idea what was occurring. How could she have let that happen? She must have deserved it, she thought.

Juliana's heart was pounding by the time her feet hit the linoleum and she fled behind the kitchen wall, out of Barney's sight. She struggled to choke down the fear before it welled into tears. She looked frantically around the kitchen for her daughter. Only when she finally saw Erin, sitting by the refrigerator in her walker, did she finally take a breath. Erin reached up toward Juliana with her small fingers. Juliana wondered how she was going to protect her daughter from this. She had not even been able to protect herself. She picked up Erin and held her close.

Juliana's mom walked into the kitchen and looked in the pot as Juliana sat feeding macaroni to Erin at the table. "Macaroni again. Why do you always insist on buying that?"

"It's Erin's favorite, and besides, it was all we could afford," Juliana replied without looking up.

"Well then, why don't you get that baby daddy of yours to help out?" her mother retorted. "If you had any sense you would have been able to pick a man who would stick around. Instead you went and made a baby with the most useless one you could find, just because you could."

Juliana didn't look up. Her mother knew full well that Erin's father had disappeared from Juliana's life the second there was a pink line on her pregnancy test. Juliana didn't blame him. They certainly had not planned on this happening, and she might have run too if she could have. Still, her mother insisted on telling her at least once a week about her poor choice in men. Juliana kept quiet. Her silence was the fastest way to end the conversation. She had never been able to tell her mother what had happened to her. It wasn't safe. Her mother would think she was as dirty as she felt, or worse. So she shut her mouth, dropped her eyes lower, and dug the baby spoon in the macaroni again for Erin.

Juliana felt herself slip another rung lower on the rope ladder she pictured dangling off a cliff. Erin bounced her legs against the high chair and looked up at Juliana with big dark eyes. Juliana looked back at the person bringing her the most happiness in the world and brought another spoonful of macaroni to her little mouth. She wanted so desperately to be the mom Erin deserved, to be able to protect her from the memories that haunted Juliana, and yet she felt she was miserably failing to do that.

The bell rang, jolting Juliana in her chair. It was fifth period and she had fallen asleep again. Math used to be her favorite, but she had fallen asleep in class so many times that when she opened her books at night she didn't know what the symbols meant, never mind how to stumble through the problems. Erin had a cold again, which meant Juliana had been up all night for the third night in a row while Erin cried and fussed.

"Put your homework on my desk on your way out," Mr. Jackson said.

Juliana hadn't even looked at her homework last night. It didn't matter. She wouldn't have understood it anyway, she thought. There was no way she could pass ninth grade as far as she could tell. So why bother? She was so tired she couldn't think about anything but sleep. Juliana watched everyone else get up and tried to walk behind a group of people so that Mr. Jackson wouldn't see her.

"Juliana," she heard him say as she slipped out the door. She pretended she didn't hear him and rushed down the hall before he had a chance to catch up with her.

Juliana felt ashamed in front of most other teachers. "Did you hear she had a baby two years ago? She's another one of those girls who's making irresponsible choices and wasting her life," she had overheard her English teacher, Mrs. Richardson, say to another teacher one day as she walked past the teachers' lounge. Mrs. Richardson wore makeup caked so thick sometimes Juliana was amazed she could open her mouth to talk, and she was ordained with pearl earrings, pink suits, and an ostentatious diamond on her finger that probably cost as much as a house in Detroit. She drove in from the suburbs. Juliana hated having to sit there and listen to those teachers.

When they found out that she had a baby, they started to treat her differently. She felt exposed. As if the whole world knew that she had had sex and everyone was there to judge her. But no one knew how it felt. No one knew that her body went numb with fear. No one knew that all she could think of were the times when she had fought and fought fruitlessly to get that first man off her without ever succeeding.

When one of the teachers got pregnant this year, they threw parties and celebrated. Some even talked about how wonderful it was. Why did they treat Juliana like she had committed a felony for the same thing? They talked about how hard it was for that teacher to be up late at night taking care of her baby. Yet Juliana's report cards said she was irresponsible for not getting her homework done, when she too had been up all night taking care of her baby.

Mr. Jackson was different. He never made Juliana feel that way. He was the only man she had ever felt comfortable around. His class was orderly. No one spoke out of turn when he was in the room. He was six feet three inches tall, slim, and had deep black skin. He dressed in a suit most days. Mr. Jackson had grown up in Detroit. Juliana didn't know any other teachers who had grown up in Detroit. The first day of class he had stood in front of the room and told them, "It is possible, but you are going to have to work harder than every other student out there if you want to make it."

No one had ever said those words to Juliana—or, as far as she knew, to anyone in her school. Most teachers arrived in Detroit excited and energetic and within six months gave up any hope of improving things. To Juliana, that also meant giving up hope on her and the other students. Mr. Jackson never stopped until everyone in the classroom understood the lesson. He never made anyone feel embarrassed.

When Juliana had failed her first test after staying up all night with Erin, he had quietly pulled her aside after school, sat down in a student's desk next to her, and gone through the problems one at a time until she understood. He never acted like she wasn't smart enough to understand. No one had ever said that it was possible before, that there was something else to think and dream about. No teacher had ever treated her like she was worthwhile. She hadn't understood at first when he sat teaching her after school, until she finally realized that he really thought she could understand. She had done better in his class than she had done in any class since she got pregnant.

That was months ago, though. That was before she sat in the bathtub nightly, wondering if ending her life would be better, and before the events of her past started lurking in every corner of her mind. Now she couldn't find the energy to get through Mr. Jackson's class. Even his message, running through all his teaching and lectures, that anything was possible, couldn't touch the emptiness inside her. So she avoided eye contact with him and ran out the door when he tried to catch up with her. She knew he had noticed that she was sleeping in every class and she hadn't done any of her homework, but all she wanted to do was avoid him.

That day, as Juliana headed out of the school to jump on the bus with her backpack over one shoulder, Mr. Jackson sat waiting for her on the front steps. He caught her eyes before she had a chance to avoid him.

"Juliana," Mr. Jackson called from the step.

"Oh, Mr. Jackson," Juliana replied as she slowed her pace and walked in his direction. There was no escaping this time. She stared at her worn sneakers so that she wouldn't have to look at his eyes. She couldn't believe he had caught her.

"You are not alone. Please call." He placed a card in her hand, and she glanced at it briefly. It was a bright-orange card that said something about a teen clinic on it.

"I don't have any health insurance. I can't afford this." Juliana tried to hand the card back to him.

"It's free. You deserve this. Please call." Before Juliana could protest, Mr. Jackson folded her hand around the card, stood up, and walked back into the building. She wasn't quite sure what this meant or what she was supposed to do. She stashed the card in the back pocket of her jeans and headed for the bus.

That night, instead of sitting in the tub, Juliana sat on the edge of the bed she shared with Erin, flipping the card over in her hand. Barney was downstairs again, drinking away the last of their food money. Erin was still sick, her mother was upset with her again, and Juliana felt the emptiness creeping over her. She had never asked for help before. That was what wealthy people did. She wondered why Mr. Jackson thought this would be for her. What was a teen clinic? Juliana got up, intending to throw the card in the trash, but paused, took a deep breath, and picked up her phone.

Juliana sat on the table where the nurse asked her to sit and the paper crinkled underneath her. There were drawings on the wall of trees and lakes. The walls were bright blue with grapefruit trim, not the office beige she had pictured. She tried to plan out what she would say, but she had no idea.

She had made up a story about a cough to the woman on the phone. Her hands were sweaty and left wet marks on the paper underneath her.

After an eternity of her stomach tying knots in itself, a woman with graying blond hair in a loose ponytail down her back walked in the door. She was calm. It felt like she had time. She introduced herself with her first name, Annie, but her badge told Juliana she was her doctor. Juliana had pictured someone stiff and proper, but this woman was everything but rigid. She wore a sporty skirt and shoes that looked like she was about to climb a mountain. She was practical. She sat down and just said, "Hello."

Juliana let one of the knots in her stomach release. She hadn't been sure she would tell this women anything, but in the middle of talking about a cough she didn't have, the story started to unfold. First, school. Then Erin. Then the bathtub. Juliana didn't know where it came from, but the story flowed out of her.

Juliana expected Annie to back off or call her crazy and walk out of the room as soon as she mentioned her emptiness and the way she wished she could just slip beneath the water and end her life. Instead, Annie reached out and took Juliana's hand in both of hers. She looked Juliana right in the eye and waited.

Then the secret Juliana had never told anyone came pouring out with the tears she had never let herself cry. She talked about the first man who had abused her, when she was five. How she had never felt well since. How she was petrified that the same thing would happen to Erin and she wouldn't be able to protect her. Through everything Annie sat and patiently listened. Juliana had feared that if she told someone, they would think she was as indecent as she felt, as undeserving of life. But Annie didn't grimace or shy away. She listened carefully and never let go of Juliana's hand. When Juliana's story slowed and she paused, Annie looked right at her again. "It is not your fault, and you are not alone."

Annie had been trying to get Juliana to come to her group for months.

Juliana trusted Annie at this point, but she wasn't sure about the idea of talking in a group. She still hadn't told anyone else. The idea of sitting in a quiet room and sharing her story with other people her age was too overwhelming.

Instead, Juliana came up with a million excuses. She had to take care of Erin, she needed to do homework, her mom needed her to cook dinner. Juliana knew that Annie saw right through these excuses, but the doctor kept waiting patiently. Finally, at the end of an appointment in the early spring, Annie simply said, "I'll see you Saturday at nine. Wear clothes that can get dirty, and bring Erin." Annie left the room before Juliana could protest.

Juliana showed up that Saturday in torn jeans and an old T-shirt with Erin on her hip. She had no idea what to expect. "Good," was all Annie said when she met her in the front of the clinic. "Grab two shovels from that pile and come with me." Juliana grabbed the shovels and headed off behind Annie. They walked two blocks down the street from the clinic and stopped at a yellow-and-pink picket fence lined with the first crocuses and daffodils of spring. Juliana couldn't believe that this had been right down the street. She had never seen it before. There was a group of other girls all her age waiting by the gate. Annie handed each of them a box of seeds and opened the gate. Inside, waiting to be planted, were eight garden beds.

"Hey, it must be your first day here," a girl standing next to Juliana said. She was tall and dark. Her hair was tied with a band and spread in a tall fro above her hair band. She was one of the most beautiful girls she had ever seen, Juliana thought. The girl stuck out her hand. "I'm Olivia. Welcome. Let me show you."

Olivia poured a small pile of seeds into Juliana's hand and one into Erin's too. Olivia knelt in front of the first bed, drew a line in the dark earth with her finger, then poked seeds into the earth, one at a time and a few inches apart. "These are peas. We'll build them bean poles to grow up once they start to sprout. Go ahead, I'll show you how." Juliana hesitated.

"Aaron," Olivia called. A small boy came running over from the next bed. She whispered something in his ear. He ran over and reached up for Erin. Juliana set Erin on the ground, the seeds still wrapped in her little hand. Aaron took her other hand and pulled her over to the nearest bed. She looked up at Juliana, who nodded to go ahead, and together the children ran to the next garden bed. "Come on," Olivia said, burying both her hands right in the dirt.

Juliana put the seeds in a pile and sunk her hands into the soil beside Olivia's. It was moist and warm. It felt good. Juliana had never seen a real garden before. Juliana still wasn't sure how these dried seeds made the greenish brown, round vegetables she had seen on her lunch trays at school, but she followed Olivia's lead. She drew straight lines in the earth, safely deposited the seeds in their own holes to the depth of her first finger joint, and gently covered them with soil.

That day they planted peas, carrots, lettuce, kale, chard, squash, and nasturtiums, all of the early-spring crops. Erin learned alongside Juliana, soaking up the first Michigan sun of spring, covering her little fingers in dirt and giggling with joy at the worms she uncovered. By the end of the day, Juliana's nails were black, her jeans were covered in earth, and her muscles were sore. She felt wonderful.

That night Juliana helped Erin in and out of the bath and then jumped in herself. For the first time in months the water felt warm and welcoming. The thought of slipping underneath it seemed so distant and different in her mind. Instead she let it soothe her sore muscles, rejoiced in its warmth, and jumped out when she was done to bring Erin to bed.

"Mama, fun," Erin said as they climbed into bed together. It was the first time she had said the word "fun." Juliana smiled then tickled Erin until she shrieked and giggled. Erin snuggled up against Juliana, and after months of not sleeping, Juliana slept well.

By the end of the summer, Juliana was an expert in sugar snap peas, lettuce, squash, tomatoes, peppers, flowers, greens, and more vegetables than she had ever known existed. On weekends in the steamy summer heat of Michigan, Annie helped them harvest the sun-kissed bounty of their garden. Together they cooked a meal in her big open kitchen. Juliana learned how to cook everything that grew in their garden.

Aaron and Erin became as close as siblings. Together they became experts in all the bugs in the garden. They captured fireflies and put jars of them on the table before Annie made them set them loose again. They sat in front of Annie's big windows and watched with excitement and giggles as summer thunderstorms broke the heat of the day.

Olivia and Juliana spent their afternoons side by side. They rarely talked about the things that had happened to them, but they knew that when they did, the other unconditionally understood. That summer, together they mixed salad dressings, spread dough for pizza with veggie toppings, cut strawberries, and whipped cream by hand to dip the strawberries in. Annie's kitchen became Juliana's haven. There, she felt safe and loved.

When she finally built up the courage, Juliana brought home the first food from the garden. She started with butternut squash. One night, while her mother was still at work, she peeled, cut, and steamed the squash until it was a deep rich orange. She served it on plates of rice, with sage from the garden cooked in butter, and held her breath until her mother came home.

Her mother looked weary at first. Juliana remembered her first time eating fresh vegetables, how different it tasted, and reminded herself to be patient. Still, she was nervous. This was something she had built on her own. Part of her feared allowing her mother into this world, this part of herself, which was independent and proud. To her surprise, her mother sat down at the table next to her and instead of lighting a cigarette, folded a napkin on her lap. Her mother had so rarely treated her with respect that she was touched when her mother put a small piece of squash in her mouth and ate it quietly. The house was silent for what seemed like forever to Juliana. Finally, her mother looked up at her. "Juliana, this is delicious."

That night when she climbed out of the bath, Juliana paused and looked in the mirror. She was surprised by what she saw in front of her. Her shoulders had become broad and strong. Her face was filled out. Her body looked elegant and proud. Her hair was free above her head, the way it had always wanted to be. For the first time in her life, she looked in the mirror and saw someone beautiful.

▨

Juliana stood up from her folding chair as the principal called her name. For the first time she noticed the weight of the graduation robe on her shoulders. She lifted her head, looked out over the stage, and took her first step across it. As she stepped forward, the principal stood aside and Mr. Jackson stood up from behind him and took his place. He handed Juliana a bouquet of tulips, daffodils, irises, and jewel nasturtiums, then leaned forward and kissed her softly on the cheek, over the scar that she had been ashamed of for so long. He reached for the diploma the principal handed to him, and as he placed it in her hands, he said, "You made it possible. You worked harder than any student I have ever taught, and Juliana, you shine like the sun."

▨

Juliana looked out over the classroom of students. After all these years, when she stood in front of a class to teach about abuse, the memories still tried to creep in and haunt her. She was amazed at how deep those wounds had cut. But she acknowledged them calmly and they were soon overcome by the image of the beauty she had found within herself and the other women she had met on her journey.

Juliana talked to the class frankly and honestly. It was her mission to make young people aware. To make sure that no one would have to suffer the isolation and fear that she had lived with for so long. As she spoke, one girl held her gaze firmly on the marks on her table. Her shoulders slumped and her head hung on her neck. Her name tag read "June," and she would be the next young woman Juliana and Erin would ask to join them in their garden. Together they would help Detroit flourish again into a new Paris of the West.

16
We All Fight

Charlie Speicher

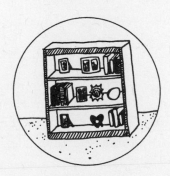

"We All Fight" introduces the complex interactions of structural violence and health outcomes. Living on the Blackfeet Reservation, Jim Two Ravens has faced many struggles in his life, such as an absent father, an incarcerated mother, and a lack of social support to attend school and think about his future. Living in rural poverty, as many do on the "rez," can contribute to many health issues, from drug and alcohol abuse to the effects of violence. In many cases, these health concerns are associated with the stress of poverty, which over many years can contribute to poor coping behaviors. Although there are many positive attributes of people living on reservations in the United States, such as a strong cultural identity, this story highlights how living in extreme poverty can contribute to violence and poor health outcomes, in this case injury. Jim's experiences place him in a difficult situation that he could not have foreseen, which results in damage to his health and his future despite his best efforts to move beyond the situation to which he was born.

Julia brushed her arm across his back as she played the slots at the casino. Jim Two Ravens didn't usually talk to Napikwans, the word for white people in the Blackfeet language. But this girl was particularly beautiful; he let down his guard and responded to her advance. "Oops," she said as she flipped back her hair.

Jim watched her walk away, and their eyes met more than once throughout the night. Jim was at a rodeo event—a benefit dinner at the casino in Browning, Montana; Julia's family was in the casino business. At the end of the night, Julia approached him.

"Will you be in Great Falls next weekend?" she asked.

"Yeah," he said with a smile. "See you there?"

"Jim, did you find the TV remote?" Leroy yelled out the broken window. Jim looked up to see his cousin staring at him wearing only his underwear. "Everyone is tough around here," Jim huffed as he shook his head at his cousin.

Jim was in the alley behind his house on the 700 block of Browning's Low Rent district. He'd been looking through the trash to find a missing TV remote for an hour and was beginning to feel chilled. There was garbage everywhere: in the cans, behind the cans, and all over the bumpy two-track road that stretched behind the strung-together houses. Dilapidated fences separated the rows and rows of Bureau of Indian Affairs (BIA) housing in Low Rent.

The dealers were all in this part of town. The elders condemned the activity, and not all areas of Browning were like this, but Low Rent thrived on an outlaw pulse. Jim had lived there all of his life, and he knew that the poorest of the poor lived on the 700 block. Many of the houses were like Jim's, run-down and shared by multiple generations of families.

Family trees in Indian country were complicated, and Jim's family tree was no exception. Jim knew that the word *family* held many meanings on the rez. Jim was raised by his grandparents, and many of his aunties and uncles adopted their nieces and nephews, Jim's siblings. People took care of their families.

"I can't find it, Leroy," Jim called out. "It's not here."

Jim had quit school over a year ago, and since then he had spent most of his days like this, passing time with Leroy. After his mom went to prison, things at home became really difficult and his family seemed to disband in different directions. Leroy started selling meth and people were always moving through his house. His oldest brother moved to somewhere on the Crow reservation with a woman he ran around with. His two sisters each had two babies, and neither of them had a consistent man in their lives. Soon after his mother was incarcerated, Jim's grandparents died in a house fire. Their death certificates named smoke inhalation as the official cause of death, but everyone knew they were probably drunk.

Jim didn't plan to quit school, but he had had enough. He was caught with chewing tobacco in algebra and then knocked out a classmate later that week. He deserved it, Jim thought. And I'd do it again if I saw him now.

"If you can't find it, it's not there," Leroy said. "Somebody jacked it."

As Jim headed inside his house, a cold breeze blew snow off the roof tires and into his eyes. Glacier Park and the Rocky Mountains, the Backbone, as the elders called it, loomed like a white monolith in the west. He looked up at the hovering mountains and breathed out; he always found some solace in their vastness. His father used to tell him stories of the mountains and how his ancestors would take shortcuts over high mountain passes to raid enemy tribes on the west side. The mountains served as an abundant source of game and shelter in the old days. He liked to think about how his people were before the reservation came to be.

Jim entered the house and dropped down onto the couch across from his cousin. He stretched out his arms and legs out in front of him and looked at the bookcase, adjacent to the couch. The bookcase had long been the focal point of the house and was the only piece of furniture anyone cared for. The couches were full of stains and holes, and the coffee table had been broken during a fight and tossed through a window five years before. The bookcase wasn't nice by white folks' standards, but all of Jim's family was represented in the photo collection adorning each shelf. Before Jim's mom went to jail, she had compiled the family photos her mother had given her. Placing those photos in the bookcase was the only thing Jim had seen his mother work hard at in her life. And now she was in prison for at least seven years.

Of the seventy-three cousins in the photos on the bookcase, Jim estimated that maybe half were dead. Just last year, six of his cousins had been killed in one drunk-driving crash alone. It didn't really hurt Jim to look at the pictures of his dead cousins. He rarely thought of them. In fact, Jim never heard anyone mention death in his family. All Jim knew about death was that he wasn't supposed to cry in public if he was at a funeral. And these days it seemed as though he was at a funeral every week.

Jim stretched his feet out before him and raised his arms above his head, clenching his jaw. By his count, he had been in twenty to twenty-three fistfights in his life. He'd won about twelve of them, and winning mattered. He was known for his strength in Browning; it was how he earned respect. Jim knew that fighters could do whatever they wanted, as long as they didn't cross paths with someone even tougher. It would be "OK," the Blackfeet would say, if the men kept their fists off their women. But they didn't. Most families in Browning had histories of domestic violence and spousal abuse, and his was no different.

"How you gonna get there?" Leroy asked Jim, as he picked through the small crystallized bags of "teenths" from the cushion next to him, filing them away in a decrepit envelope.

"These guys I talked to the other night are gonna drive me if I give 'em gas money. William Black Weasel's cousin or somethin'." His mind wandered to what would happen that night. He figured he'd hitchhike back from Great Falls, depending on how long he stayed with Julia.

"You sure that's a good idea? If it's William's family, they're probably drunks and thieves," Leroy said. He was serious. It was difficult for Jim to understand how Leroy would worry about him since Leroy was well aware that Jim was plenty experienced in interacting with addicts, given Leroy's current occupation. But that was exactly why Leroy was concerned. The dealers in town often knew which families struggled the most.

"I hear bad things about that family, and I have seen William blow up out of nowhere," he muttered. "They're rough. Just watch yourself if you ride with those guys."

Jim nodded at his cousin, lost in his own nervousness about the date. It was the first one he'd ever had with a girl off the rez. Anticipating what she might think of him, Jim had found a job earlier that week just for the occasion. Well, not a full-time job. He and his uncle Marlo took the old Chevy into the mountains near East Glacier and got a load of wood. Sometimes the local doctors would buy a load if you brought it by the hospital around the time their shift ended. And dependable old Dr. Warren came through again—he even gave Jim and Marlo a twenty-dollar tip each. Coupled with his take from the wood, Jim had in his pocket the largest amount of money he'd ever had at one time. He was ready for the date.

"When you gonna leave?"

"Like an hour." Jim's thoughts drifted to Julia. He wondered if he would be able to sleep with her tonight. A wry smile took over his face.

✸

Two hours later, Jim was far from smiling. He had felt the pain of broken ribs before. Twice, actually. But that didn't come close to the pain Jim now felt in his side. They'd stabbed him and kicked him in the face. He felt a searing pain in his lower right jaw that went down to his neck.

Jim tried desperately to sort out what had just occurred, but everything blurred together. He saw a flash of the person who had stabbed him, the guy who had picked him up. They had taken a detour en route and picked up two other guys that Jim didn't know and, at some point, they all decided to rob Jim. They pulled over to the side of Interstate 15 and began yelling at him. He felt a blow to his head and blacked out. But the next thing he remembered was standing over his friend's cousin, who was bloodied and lying by the car, pleading his innocence to Jim.

Jim climbed into the driver's seat of the car and floored it. He didn't know where he was going—he just needed to get away. His breathing deepened as he went over the events of the night. He began to hyperventilate as he drifted to the side of the road, crashing over the rumble strips with reckless abandon. Luckily the strips snapped him into the present and he jerked the wheel to the left. Jim straightened his trajectory and began to pick up the pace.

Lights and signs flashed by, but Jim didn't recognize where he was. He tried to calculate what was happening, but his thoughts raced.

Did I kill him? he thought. He was moaning last I remember, so at least he was alive then.

Up ahead was a sign that read "Great Falls—13 Miles." The sign brought him back to the present and Jim remembered why he was going there in the first place: Julia. Jim knew other people in Great Falls, but they were all connected to Browning. Sometimes when you are in trouble with one Indian, you're soon in trouble with the whole tribe, Jim thought. He accelerated, knowing he had to get to the mall to find Julia. Maybe she would help him.

The miles rapidly ticked by as Jim's fear set in. He took inventory of his options. He'd have to fight more people over this. There was no way around that. There's always an older brother or cousin or associate or even acquaintance of someone you beat up who's ready to go next. Jim's friend William certainly wouldn't be happy.

All of a sudden, Jim saw bright lights in his mirrors. The red-and-blue lights grew until they were right on his tail. Jim's panic took over. No longer did the numbing pain in his ribs feel like anything. And no more could Jim feel the blood pooling in the creases of his jeans on his waist. All he felt was fear. The helpless realization that he was in big trouble enveloped his thoughts and consumed his awareness.

"Pull over!" the officer yelled from his speakers on top of the car. "Pull over immediately!"

Go! Jim's internal senses screamed. Drive now! Jim didn't know where that command came from, but he decided to follow it. He floored it.

Jim swerved onto the rumble strips again but corrected the wheels and sped off. This must have taken the cop by surprise, because he soon fell behind. Jim roared over the asphalt like a freight train and pulled hard to the right as he saw the two-track ranch access road appear as an exit from the highway.

The patrolman quickly gained on Jim as the Impala began to hit the ruts in the center of the road. As long as I don't crack the oil pan, I can make it, Jim thought. The two-track road soon came to a T and broke left and right onto County Road 42, a gravel frontage road of the interstate. Jim turned left and headed toward the lights of Great Falls. The lights bled into the prairies and dotted the landscape and it was difficult to see where the night sky and the bright stars in it ended. Jim had the accelerator fully depressed when the engine began to sputter. He looked down to see the fuel gauge at empty.

Jim's heart sank to his chest as the car burned the last of the gas fumes away and drifted to a halt. An overwhelming sense of finality engulfed him, and he placed his hands on his lap and glanced in the mirror. The lights were stopped behind him now, and a shadowy figure was shouting at him.

The figure was soon at Jim's window and tugging at the door handle. As the car door opened, Jim locked eyes with the highway patrolman. The officer's mouth was moving but Jim couldn't hear what he was saying. The 9 mm he held caught Jim's attention. There were more red-and-blue lights at the scene and more people shouting at him. Jim was now circled by shadowy figures as the patrolman pulled the Taser from his waist and aimed at Jim's midsection.

Jim finally turned his face to the officer's and slowly muttered, "It wasn't my fault."

He stood up and approached the young officer. The officer took a step backward and shouted but Jim didn't stop. He fired the Taser and Jim's body tensed and limply crumbled to the ground.

17

Nelson's Soweto

Emily Mendenhall

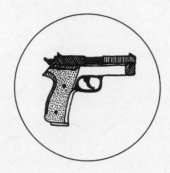

"Nelson's Soweto" discusses the role of violence in Nelson's community. Nelson is a teenager living in Soweto, a township in Johannesburg, South Africa. Soweto is both technologically advanced, with 95 percent cell phone coverage, and structurally flawed, with many people living in shacks without access to plumbing or flushable toilets. Gun violence is common in his neighborhood, and his brother died as a result of cross fire two years ago. His parents died from AIDS when he was young, a common occurrence because one in four people in Soweto are HIV positive. His grandmother, who is raising him, can't afford to move to a wealthier area of the city, so they continue to live in an unsafe neighborhood. This story describes how the recent loss of a close friend to gun violence brings up the realities of the threat of such violence and the problems that breed violence among young men in Soweto. The history of apartheid, and its laws against people of different racial and ethnic backgrounds living and working side by side, and increasing inequalities in current-day unemployment, have contributed to the high prevalence of such violence in Nelson's community.

Nelson ran through the moonlit street and turned the corner at an all-too-familiar curb. Every time he passed this curb, a memory flashed into his consciousness. Today he buried it and kept running. Matimba was close on his heels, and he did not want his friend to catch up after the prank.

"I'm gonna get you, Nelson!" cried Matimba. Nelson couldn't stop laughing and finally, grabbing a steel post, turned around to face Matimba and to hold himself up as his laughter intensified. "What, you think it's funny?"

"The look on your face, Matimba!" Matimba's face softened, and his angry frown turned to laughter. Nelson put his hand on Matimba's shoulder and they laughed together before they turned around to walk back to their friends.

Gunshots sounded relatively close to where they were standing. It was not an uncommon sound in their neighborhood, so Nelson and Matimba continued walking back to their friends, unfazed.

"But if you put a spicy hot pepper in my bunny chow ever again, you're really gonna get it." Nelson just chuckled as the two friends walked back the four blocks they had traveled as a result of a hot, spicy bite in Matimba's favorite sandwich.

When they arrived back to where their friends had been standing—in front of their favorite neighborhood market store—no one was to be found. Instead, Nelson saw Jackson's blue Tommy Hilfiger sweat shirt lying on the ground and blood ten feet away from it. He looked up at Matimba, who had a worried look on his face. Without exchanging words, the boys turned around and began walking the six blocks to their respective residences, Nelson with Jackson's sweat shirt in his hand.

🔲

In the morning, Nelson received a text message from Jackson: "Bad nite. Where did u go?" Nelson already knew what had happened. The *tsotsis* (gang members) had been terrorizing his friends for years, in addition to the rest of the neighborhood. Two months ago, Nelson was beaten up so badly that he had to go to Baragwanath Hospital to stitch up a cut on his upper lip and a slice on his forehead. Afterward, Mama Hunadi, his grandmother, took him to Kentucky Fried Chicken for his favorite crispy chicken strips—a special treat.

"You don't deserve this crispy chicken." Her words were like cold ice at the foot of the bed in the midst of winter. "You know what Rhulani went through with those boys. They're just gonna come back for you. You're out in the night in their territory. They own those streets, boy. And next time it's going to be guns, not knives. Why don't you listen to me? Use your nights for studying inside the house, not passing time in the streets."

Nelson gave her respect and continued to listen as she lectured him. Ashamed, he kept his eyes down at his plate.

"You know I had the same talk with Rhulani and now he can't enjoy this fresh chicken with me," she said. "You just think about that some, Nelson."

Her words were ironed into his memory. But only last night had they really set in. Nelson continued to lie in his bed, his mind racing and his heart unsettled. He didn't want to cause more trouble, but he didn't want to spend his days and nights locked inside, behind the iron gates and security alarm, like he was in jail. He had to live his life with his friends. But his grandmother's words were never louder than they were that morning, with Jackson and his friends in trouble.

"You up?" Mama Hunadi asked as she popped her head into Nelson's bedroom.

Nelson moved his head to face her. "Yeah," he said sheepishly, knowing she already knew more than he did. He looked over at his little brother, who still slept soundly. He threw on a hooded sweat shirt and got out of bed.

"You weren't there last night. Where were you? Where was Matimba? The other boys got it bad; they are at Baragwanath gettin' fixed up. Michael might not make it."

Nelson looked down at his hands and pushed back a lump in his throat. "Yeah. We weren't there."

"You better be telling me the truth, boy. You escaped it this time, but if God Almighty loves me, you will tell me the truth. I can't take this anymore. You weren't in your bed until late."

"We weren't there, Mama Hu. We weren't there."

She seemed unsatisfied but left to finish preparing breakfast. Ever since Rhulani died, she had prepared his favorite fried eggs every Saturday morning before she began her housework. Even when eggs were too expensive, she sacrificed other household needs so she could purchase eggs. This Saturday was no different.

Nelson sat at the table with his head in his hands, fighting back tears. Last night, he had met up with his friends at their usual spot, in front of their favorite store, the one that makes the best bunny chow in the neighborhood. It wasn't different from other nights. But recently, the tsotsis had gotten more confident, more active. He felt that something was brewing like it had two years ago.

"What was it like when Rhulani was shot, Mama Hu? What did it feel like in the neighborhood?" He knew he was treading into dangerous territory, because his grandmother often got upset when he brought up his brother. His grandmother had experienced great loss over the past ten years. First, she lost her daughter and son-in-law to AIDS. Despite her grief and shame, because AIDS was very stigmatized in South Africa, she took in the three boys to raise them on her own. She didn't speak of her daughter's death for three years. Because Nelson had been so small, he didn't understand until much later why his parents had died. Then, two years ago, Rhulani was shot dead during a burglary. Rhulani wasn't involved, but he was shot in the cross fire when tsotsis were breaking into a neighbor's house.

Violence was common in Soweto, the South Western Townships. This was predominantly the home of black South Africans who had been relocated and displaced numerous times through the settlement of Johannesburg. It was the home of South Africa's most famous revolutionary and first democratic president, Nelson Mandela, but it was also famous for its high rates of gun violence. After Rhulani was shot, Mama Hu put up iron bars on their windows and installed an iron door to protect her family from tsotsis. She buried her feelings in making a fortress of her house.

"It was heatin' up," Mama Hunadi said. "The tsotsis had more confidence. Our next door neighbor was robbed. She lost everything. I was nervous every time someone passed our house on the street after dark. Even in the daylight, people got robbed by tsotsis. What's worse, I knew most of those young men." She gave a deep sigh. "We didn't fight apartheid to now live in fear of our young men. I don't know what's to be done."

Nelson gave his grandmother soft eyes as she put a plate of fried eggs in front of him. He soaked up the gooey middle with his toast and gobbled it down. With the last bite of toast, Nelson asked, "Will you go to Bara with me? I need to check on the boys."

"Get cleaned up. I've already spoken with Michael's mother, who is there. We'll need to leave in ten minutes to catch the minibus."

"Was 2 blox away. Got back & u gone. Be at Bara in hour," Nelson texted back to Jackson.

Nelson and Mama Hunadi arrived to Baragwanath Hospital to a bustling Saturday market. He noticed Mama Hu had tucked an extra grocery bag under her arm when they left the house. "In case there is a good deal on okra," she said.

They crossed the bridge from the market over Old Potchefstroom Road to Baragwanath Hospital and Nelson felt his heart speed up. It could be me in there, he thought.

They reached reception and were frisked before they entered the hospital and headed to the Trauma Unit. When they reached the waiting room, Nelson saw that Jackson's hand was tightly bandaged but otherwise he looked all right, although somewhat tattered and disgruntled. "Michael's in surgery again," Jackson said when he saw Nelson and Mama Hunadi. "He's in his third surgery since we came in last night. He won't stop bleeding internally."

Mama Hunadi saw Michael's mother and went to comfort her.

Nelson nodded as Jackson took a deep breath to continue. "We didn't see them coming. You and Matimba ran off and we didn't even hear them. I think they were headed down the street to do a job; we were in the way. They didn't want us there. We weren't doing anything, just joking around. Michael spoke up, saying something that grabbed their attention. Juggs turned around; his eyes were cold and he looked straight at Michael and shot him. He was shot in the shoulder, the stomach, and the leg. He lost so much blood. I ran to Michael and another guy grabbed my arm, twisted my hand so badly he broke it. Pushed me on the ground hard and grabbed my shirt. Came right off."

Nelson pulled Jackson's signature blue Tommy Hilfiger sweat shirt out of his bag and handed it to him.

"Thanks," Jackson squawked through suppressed tears.

Nelson sat down next to his friend, crossed his arms across his chest, and closed his eyes as they waited for news of their friend.

One week later, everyone was dressed in white and standing in a field away from town. Michael was Zionist, so he was buried and remembered during a ceremony held outside on a hill on the outskirts of Soweto proper. Michael was thirteen and had never owned a gun, but he had held many of them. Nelson, Matimba, and Jackson huddled together, staring at the ground. No one knew what to say.

Nelson didn't know everyone at the service because he was Methodist and didn't worship with Michael. But he followed the hymns, prayers, and speeches that the people made to honor Michael's life. Mama Hu noticed him staring at people's white robes and said, "All the Zionists wear these robes to funerals, and funerals are all outside." Mama Hunadi attended the funeral as she attended all of the funerals of young people in their neighborhood. She turned back to the ceremony that took the whole day, but for Nelson the funeral seemed to take only minutes. He was lost in the energy of the singing and drumming, and sorrow of burying his friend.

Nelson walked home with Mama Hunadi. She walked a bit ahead of Nelson and he was glad to have some space to clear his head and breath after such an intense day. She seemed to see he was distressed.

After some time, Mama Hunadi spoke, as she often did, words of wisdom. "I remember a day when we fought together, Nelson. It was us against them. We fought apartheid, racial injustice, together. There was an energy in the community that you could feel and we believed in changing our lives."

Not in the mood for a motherly speech, Nelson held his chin to his chest and walked on just a foot behind his grandmother.

"When Nelson Mandela, your namesake, was released from prison in 1990, we knew things would be different. Madiba [Mandela's nickname] was a real leader who unified our people."

She picked up her pace, and so did Nelson.

"Four years later, when Madiba became president of the new South Africa, one where white and black people could walk together equally in a country where previously race divided us, we were determined to have access to education and justice. I knew things would be different. And they were."

Nelson continued to walk forward with his head down, tracing each step with his eyes.

"But things have changed in the last ten years. Things have not gotten better for us here. The Black Diamonds, the political elite, have grown rich. They are sitting on their coffers in fancy homes, driving fancy cars, eating fancy foods. But here in Soweto and other townships, many that are worse off than us, the health centers are still not stocked. The roads are not paved. Sanitation is not available for everyone. The schools are not the same here as they are in the northern suburbs of Johannesburg. This is not yet a nation where equality reigns."

Nelson picked up his pace, with his ears perked up. He knew how she felt but did not completely understand.

"It is a country that is still deeply divided," she continued. "Maybe not completely by race like it once was. But it is divided by money—who has money and who doesn't. Greed for growing one's bank account drives these young men who are not in school to violence. That is why we buried Michael today."

Mama Hunadi continued with her head high, eyes sharp as nails. "If the boys were in school. If there were more jobs. If there were more opportunities for young boys in the neighborhood. Then, there would be fewer guns, less violence, less death. Rhulani would still be here. He was a smart boy. He would be going to university or technical school. He would have made something of himself. He would have made me proud."

Nelson walked with his grandmother in silence for the thirty minutes more it took them to walk home from the funeral. They both knew that Michael's death reminded them of losing Rhulani. When they were only a few blocks from home, they passed the curb where Rhulani had fallen only two years before. The same curb that Nelson had passed only one week before when Matimba chased him for a prank that might have saved his life.

"This is where I was, Mama Hu. When Michael was shot. I was right here."

Mama Hunadi turned to her grandson, her eyes full of tears. "He is protecting his brother still. You be better, boy. You be better."

Mama Hunadi grasped her grandson's elbow tightly as they hastened home. Nelson had never felt closer to her, or to his brother's memory.

18
The Grove

Suzanne Farrell Smith

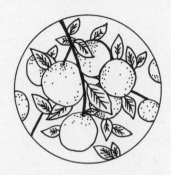

"The Grove" is the story of Kimberly, who at twelve years old discovers the ugly secret of human trafficking at the south Florida home and orange groves of her mother's best friend. It is estimated that between six hundred thousand and eight hundred thousand people every year are forced or compelled to leave their home countries and work elsewhere. These people are trafficked across international borders. Over fifteen thousand of them end up in the United States, where they find themselves at the mercy of the employers the United Nations refers to as modern-day slave owners. Trafficked people are forced to work in several industries, including prostitution, selling or transporting illegal arms or drugs, manufacturing, and agriculture. Although trafficked victims often experience interpersonal violence, "The Grove" is an example of structural violence, as trafficked victims often live and work in unsanitary conditions, are made to work nonstop for little or no pay, and receive no health care. Health problems abound, from communicable diseases such as STIs (like HIV and AIDS) to psychological trauma and malnourishment. Kimberly's discovery demonstrates how access to even basic health care could help trafficked victims with chronic illnesses.

"Stop right there, Kimberly. Don't make me come over and stop you myself."

Kimberly knew all too well the stern tone in her mother's voice.

"Come on, Mom," Kimberly said, a little too sharply. She turned to face the patio, where her mother sat on a chair with her legs crossed, one sandal dangling from her upturned toes. Kimberly offered a slight smile to soften her attitude. If there was anything her mother couldn't stand, it was a bad attitude, and Kimberly wasn't up for an argument.

Kimberly was twelve years old. She and her mother were on their monthly Saturday trip to visit friends of her parents at their large estate. Already tall for her age, Kimberly's legs felt cramped from the long car ride.

"Mom," said Kimberly, "I just feel like a walk. Why can't I go for a little bit?"

"You're not allowed in the grove," Kimberly's mother responded. "And besides, I said so, and that should be reason enough."

The estate was a far cry from their two-bedroom apartment overlooking the Intracoastal Waterway, which separated a string of barrier islands from mainland Florida. Kimberly loved to walk along the waterway, counting the flat-bottomed fishing boats, racing bowriders, graceful sailboats, and sleek yachts as they slid by on their way to and from the Atlantic Ocean.

But today there was no boat counting. There was nothing to do here. Kimberly missed the water today. She missed her life today. She sighed and shuffled back to the patio just as their hostess, Ms. Eva, came out of the giant house with a tray of iced tea and miniature bowls full of olives and dried fruit.

The Fishers, Mr. Matt and Ms. Eva, as Kimberly had been instructed to call them, owned over two hundred acres of citrus groves. They lived in a large house on the property, which also included several outbuildings. Some, like the greenhouse, were well kept. Others, like the quarters where the farmworkers and housekeepers lived, were too far from the house for Kimberly to see what they really looked like. Of course, she wasn't allowed to venture over there to get a better look. To Kimberly, this world was completely different from hers. Besides, the Fishers had no children. Kimberly ached to do something—anything—other than sit with her mother and Ms. Eva on the patio, sipping iced tea. Her father never came on these visits. She wished she could stay home with him, but her mother liked to use the car rides to quiz Kimberly about school.

Kimberly grudgingly stretched on a recliner chair and folded her arms over her chest, staring out at the grove that seemed to her both mysterious and bright. If only she could explore it.

"Such a pity about the weather this year," Kimberly's mother said to Ms. Eva.

"The frost hasn't been all that bad, but it's still been colder than it has been in a few years. Colder temps, fewer fruits."

"What are you going to do?" asked Kimberly's mother.

"We've already done it. We took some resources out of picking and are using them for the house. It's kind of nice, though. I've been dying to update the master bathroom."

Kimberly remembered Mr. Harris, her sixth-grade teacher, explaining the word *resource* in language arts class. On the quiz, she got the spelling right, and the definition too: "something that can be used for help or support, like money or property."

But as the women drifted through a conversation about tiles that don't mildew and hurricane shutters that look attractive, Kimberly drifted too, her gaze following the narrow path between trees in the grove. Each row of trees was perfectly straight, each tree round and full with branches hanging so low that some of them touched the ground. Kimberly looked at the base of a row of trees, trying to make out the trunks, when suddenly she noticed a pair of feet. She didn't dare bolt upright and earn her mother's attention. Instead, she narrowed her eyes to focus in on those feet. They were small and bare. She hadn't seen anyone besides the house staff at Ms. Eva's. Who was this mystery person in the grove?

Next to the feet rested a white pail. Before Kimberly had a chance to guess at its contents, the feet and the pail were on the move. For a split second, Kimberly saw what looked like a young, skinny boy dart across the open lane between rows of trees, dragging the pail that seemed too heavy for him. Then, he was gone.

***

By school on Monday, Kimberly had forgotten all about the boy in the grove. She had a test, and her mother was worried about her grades—Bs mostly. Good enough for Kimberly, but her mother wanted her to earn straight As. Worse, the test was in social studies. Social studies was by far Kimberly's least favorite subject. It's not that she couldn't remember people, places, and events. It was that she spent so much time memorizing them, she didn't have enough time to really understand them. She almost always got the multiple choice questions right. She was good at diagrams and timelines. But when Mr. Harris asked questions like "How do all the branches of the American government work together to create peace and a common good?" she got flustered and her ideas spilled out, disorganized and confused. She knew the three branches of government by heart and wished that could be enough for Mr. Harris. And for her mother.

"Time's up," Mr. Harris said firmly when the period was over. Kimberly liked him and thought he was funny, but he put away his joking manner when it was time for tests. He expected his students to be prepared and to follow the rules. She dropped her pencil, not having finished the last few questions. Her mother was going to be furious. Another social studies unit that would end with a B, even a B minus.

Maybe I'll have better luck with the Civil War, she thought.

***

A month later, Kimberly and her mother were back at Ms. Eva's house. For the whole car ride, her mother grilled her about her grades, and she didn't let up, even as Ms. Eva poured them iced tea. It was always iced tea at Ms. Eva's. Kimberly let her mind wander, thinking about having orange juice for once.

"College is not that far off, Kimberly," her mother said. Ms. Eva nodded along. Kimberly tried not to listen to her mother's college talk; college seemed very far off. "It's very important that you're thinking about this now. I already took you off the volleyball team. I hope I don't have to remove you from the school play."

Mention of the play snapped Kimberly's attention back to her mother. "Mom, it's not like I don't try. Especially in social studies. It's just too much information."

"You know the material," Kimberly's mother said. "You get everything right when I quiz you. Mr. Harris says you're a bright student. I just don't understand what happens on those tests."

"I hate the way Mr. Harris asks questions!"

"That's hardly an excuse. You need to study harder next time!"

The tension between Kimberly and her mother lingered, and Kimberly retreated behind its invisible wall. Ms. Eva and Kimberly's mother started a conversation about their college. That was where they met, and they had been best friends ever since. Kimberly's mother said that college was the best thing that ever happened to her. Now she wanted Kimberly to plan for college. As her mother and Ms. Eva talked about her future education, Kimberly began to feel resentful. She decided to ignore her mother and stare off into the trees.

The boy, Kimberly remembered, and her mood lifted. *How am I going to get into that grove?*

"Mom, can I have your keys?"

"For what?"

"I just want to run back to the car," she said. But she needed a good excuse. "To get my social studies book."

"Glad to see you've changed your mind about school, honey," Kimberly's mother told her. "Get a head start on studying for the next test!"

Keys in hand, Kimberly walked to the side of the house where the cars were parked. Ms. Eva and Mr. Matt had three cars, even though there were just two of them. But Kimberly didn't stop at her mother's car. She kept walking down the driveway, along the hedgerow, until she nearly reached the street. There, she looked to make sure she couldn't be seen by the women on the patio, and turned into the grove.

The fresh, sweet smell of citrus brightened Kimberly's mood. The dirt and trees, the grass underfoot, and blue sky overhead, all made Kimberly forget her grades and her mother's disapproval. The oranges, still not ripe, varied in color from pale to dark green and looked more like limes. Soon they would ripen and turn bright orange. Mr. Matt and Ms. Eva's grove was one of the largest in south Florida, and the trees seemed to go on for miles. Preoccupied by the orange trees, Kimberly almost forgot her mission, when she saw, well along one of the rows, a white pail. It must belong to the boy, she thought. Kimberly started toward the pail and soon enough was standing eye to eye with its owner. The boy was even younger than Kimberly had thought, eight or nine, she supposed, and very skinny. His legs were covered in small scratches. His long dark hair seemed greasy and unwashed.

Kimberly's smile faded. She didn't know why, but something was wrong.

"Hi," she said. The boy didn't answer, though he opened his mouth as if to say something. Kimberly saw his teeth. They were brown and spotted. A couple were missing. The boy closed his mouth again.

Kimberly studied the boy for a few seconds, time that seemed to stretch out and become longer. The boy was the skinniest child Kimberly had ever seen. The scratches on his legs seemed normal enough at first. Kimberly also got scratched up when she played during recess. But some of the boy's scratches looked deep and dirty. Kimberly could tell they hadn't been washed, treated with a first-aid cream, and bandaged, the way her teachers and parents always did for her. And his dirty hair. Kimberly had always believed that the things her parents told her to do, like taking a bath or brushing her teeth, were things all kids had to do. How many times had she asked her parents, "Do I have to?" when they told her it was time for bath time and bed. Her own hair, short and straight, was freshly trimmed and smelled like peppermint shampoo, her favorite.

Then there were his rotting teeth. Kimberly had two cavities last year, and her dentist filled them in. She hated going to the dentist, but liked that at the end of each visit she got a new toothbrush. She went back to the dentist every few months to make sure there were no more cavities. Her front teeth were a little crooked, said her mother, who wanted Kimberly to get braces. Kimberly didn't want braces, but she'd do as her mother instructed.

Everything about this boy's appearance was different from what Kimberly knew. For a moment, she wondered why his parents and teachers didn't make him do the same things that hers did. But there was something about this boy that bothered Kimberly. She didn't want to know what else was going on in his body. She couldn't even guess at the stuff that looked sick on the inside if so much looked sick on the outside. This all passed through her mind in just a few seconds, and she quickly felt overwhelmed with sadness for the boy. She wanted to reach out to him.

"My name is Kimberly." The boy stared at her. "My mother is friends with Ms. Eva." At the name, the boy's eyes widened. He picked up his white pail. Kimberly saw a pile of green fruits with holes and bruises. They looked like they've been pecked over by birds. Before she had a chance to say anything else, the boy turned and disappeared into the grove. Kimberly stared after him for a moment, then found her way back out.

❖

"Dad, I saw a boy at Ms. Eva's house."

"Oh?"

"Yes. He was in the grove. Who do you think it was?"

"Probably a worker's kid."

"Dad, he looked kind of sick. And his teeth were brown."

"That happens sometimes. Not everyone can get to the dentist."

"He's lucky his parents don't make him go," said Kimberly a little sarcastically. But as soon as the words were out, she wished she could take them back. Remembering the boy's appearance, she thought he was anything but lucky.

Kimberly's father sighed. Then he sat down at the kitchen table and pushed back a chair with his foot, indicating Kimberly should sit down too.

"The boy is probably a worker too, Kimberly. He probably works with his family for Mr. Matt and Ms. Eva."

"But he's younger than I am!" said Kimberly.

"I know," he said, and sighed again. "Kimberly . . ." But he didn't finish. Instead, he looked down at the table and traced a line in the wood with one finger.

"Dad, I'm twelve years old. Please tell me what's going on."

Kimberly's father took a deep breath and began. "Mr. Matt and Ms. Eva go to places like Haiti and Ecuador. They go to very poor communities and convince whole families to come live with them in the United States. They tell them life will be better. But when the families get here, they have to work to pay back the debt they owe Mr. Matt and Ms. Eva for bringing them here. Only then can they leave and have the better life they've been promised."

"Is that why kids have to work too? So the family can pay back the debt faster?"

Kimberly's father was quiet for a moment, as if choosing his words carefully. "The problem is, they get paid so little, it's impossible for them ever to pay back the debt. And they don't live like we do, with nice things and plenty of food. Plus they aren't usually taught to speak English, so it would be hard for them to leave the estate. It's not a good situation."

They don't live like we do, with plenty of food, Kimberly thought. She remembered the outbuildings far from the large, beautiful house where Ms. Eva and Mr. Matt lived alone. She wondered about the unripe, badly marked fruits in the boy's pail. Suddenly Kimberly couldn't remember the boy's face, only his bony elbows, his brown, spotted teeth.

"He can't go to the dentist, can he, even if he wanted to," she said.

"No," said her father. "He can't."

A sick feeling crawled up in Kimberly's throat. "How can you let this happen, Dad? How come Mom keeps going there?"

"Some things are better left alone," he said. "It's a really sad situation.

Many places are different. Many farms treat their workers well, like part of their own families. But not Mr. Matt and Ms. Eva. This is why I don't go there anymore. Your mother isn't happy with me about it. She and Ms. Eva are best friends. Ms. Eva means the world to your mom. Still, I refuse to visit. What else can I do about it?"

It was a question Kimberly couldn't answer, either.

But as she lay in her bed that night, under her warm quilt, her washed hair still damp and making her soft pillow wet, her teeth freshly brushed, and her belly full of dinner and dessert, Kimberly didn't feel content. She felt angry. And she wondered if there was something she could do about it.

Several weeks later in social studies class, Kimberly was busy learning about the events leading up to the Civil War. Again, she memorized all the dates and facts. From 1801 to 1861 America grew rapidly. Lewis and Clark explored the western part of what is today part of the United States. Slavery expanded. Wealthy landowners had already been taking people from their homes on the continent of Africa and the islands of the Caribbean, enslaving them and forcing them to work here in the United States. When the cotton gin was invented, southern slave owners expanded slavery to pick more cotton. Then the Civil War came. Kimberly learned about the big battles and the generals. She learned about the Emancipation Proclamation, a document President Abraham Lincoln wrote to declare slavery illegal in the entire country.

And when the test came, Kimberly's mother drilled her on all the facts. Kimberly wanted this to be the unit that changed things, the test that proved to her mother, once and for all, that she was a hard worker and a good student. On the morning of the test, she ate a big breakfast and washed it down with orange juice. Then, in school, she breezed through multiple-choice and true-or-false questions. She found words in the word bank to fill in sentences. She added important events to a timeline.

But then she got to Mr. Harris's final questions and, as always, she was stuck. The very first one was "How did the Civil War end slavery in the United States?"

The question stumped Kimberly. It seemed almost like a trick question. How did the Civil War end slavery in the United States? Kimberly thought of the grove as she wrote her response to Mr. Harris:

The Civil War ended one kind of slavery in the United States. But I think slavery still happens. People still come here from other countries thinking they will have a better life but they have to work and live in bad conditions. They don't get to visit doctors and play games and have days off. I think they are like slaves. At night we sleep in comfortable beds and in the morning we eat big breakfasts and drink fresh orange juice. But there are people right here in our country, a long time after the Civil War ended, who can't do the same things we can do. The people who help make our food and nice things, but can't have any of it for themselves. These people are far away from their homelands and can't get home again. I'm not a president like Abraham Lincoln, but I will find a way to help.

When Kimberly turned in her test, she held her breath. She knew it wasn't an answer Mr. Harris would think was right. But Kimberly knew in her heart that it was right.

The next day, Mr. Harris returned the tests. Kimberly stared at the grade on the top. It was an A. Mr. Harris even wrote a note: "Kimberly, I'm very proud of you. I think you should show this test to your parents."

Her first A in social studies! But Kimberly didn't think about how proud her mother would be. Instead, she thought about what she could do to help stop what she now knew was happening at Mr. Matt and Ms. Eva's grove. She thought about how easy it could be to collect supplies like toothbrushes and toothpaste. She thought of how one visit with a nurse like the one at her school might make a big difference.

She thought that this really was the unit that changed things, and not just for her. She thought about the boy in the grove.

Cure Violence
Kathy Wollner

Cure Violence, based in Chicago, Illinois, treats violence as though it were an infectious epidemic. This means it sees violence as an infection that can spread from one person to another and believes that to decrease violence, the spread of the disease must be stopped. An epidemic means that disease exists throughout a community, in more numbers than in the past. This is true of violence in many communities, including many neighborhoods in Chicago.

Cure Violence uses three main strategies to stop this process:

1. Identify and detect: using statistics and street knowledge, figure out the most at-risk areas and individuals where work should be focused.

2. Interrupt, intervene, and reduce risk: whether mediating conflict between two people or interrupting a crisis between groups, the Cure Violence team interrupts and intervenes to prevent violent events. Staff come from the communities they represent and they know who has power, who to talk to, and how to bring down a situation before it results in bloodshed.

3. Change behavior and norms: in many communities, resolving conflict with violence is the norm. Cure Violence challenges this thinking and introduces different ways to resolve conflicts in communities.

The Cure Violence process, based on the latest research in psychology and brain science, has resulted in reductions in shootings and killings by 16 to 34 percent. The organization's ways of violence interruption and behavior change have been replicated in eleven communities in Chicago and Baltimore, resulting in large reductions in violence. This approach is now being used in many U.S. cities and some other countries, including South Africa, to prevent and reduce community violence, and in Iraq to reduce interpersonal and intertribal violence.

DISCUSSION QUESTIONS

- What do you think of comparing violence to an infectious disease? Do you think that ideas can spread just like germs do?

- Why is it important to have workers who are from the communities they are working in?

- Often communities are stuck in what's called a cycle of violence— one group of people feels wronged by another and then wrongs that group back in retaliation, and then that happens all over again. Why do you think things work this way?

- Name ways to resolve conflict without turning to violence.

- How might an organization like Cure Violence work to reduce violence in Jim's community on the Blackfeet Reservation or in Nelson's community in Soweto, South Africa?

This section's information has been adapted from Cure Violence's website. To learn more about Cure Violence and to read success stories on violence reduction, visit www.CureViolence.org.

Section V

Prevention

In the context of health, *prevention* is the act of doing something that prevents disease. It might be something that an individual does or that a community (many people) does together. In fact, an effort to prevent one disease could be completely different than an effort to prevent another disease. This might have to do with the environment in which people live, causing some diseases to be more prevalent than others. It might also have to do with what is required to prevent one disease versus another.

Prevention of disease occurs at many levels: home, neighborhood, school, primary health center, and even the community as a whole. *Primary prevention*, or prevention to keep healthy, involves efforts apart from the hospital. This is because hospitals are often used to fix problems, such as symptoms that arise once someone has become sick. This is called *secondary prevention*, where the goal is to slow or stop the progression of disease or keep an injury from causing long-term disability. *Tertiary prevention* helps people manage complicated health problems, such as those we discussed in the first section with "Dadi's Chart" and "Mai'suka, My Island."

Education is a fundamental aspect of disease prevention. If we think of disease, illness, and injury as the things we find downstream in a river, prevention means intervening upstream, at the earliest point possible to keep people healthy. Educating people about diseases common in their communities and how to prevent them, therefore, is a fundamental part of helping people stay healthy and disease free.

There are many different types of diseases, commonly divided into communicable and noncommunicable diseases. Communicable, or infectious, diseases include the common cold, the flu, and HIV. They are transmitted from one person to another in different ways. Some germs cling to our skin, which is why hand washing is important. Others are found in droplets from coughing or sneezing, which is why you must cover your mouth when you cough. Others are found only in blood, semen, or vaginal fluids, which is why condoms are important in preventing sexually transmitted infections (STIs). Noncommunicable diseases include heart disease, type 2 diabetes, cancer, depression, schizophrenia, and others diseases that are chronic. There is rarely just one reason a person has these chronic diseases; some disease-causing factors are family genes, individual behaviors, and environmental factors such as toxic waste or even the lack of safe, affordable, and healthy foods.

It is important to understand that the causes and prevention of disease differ significantly from one context to another, and from one disease to another. For example, eating well and keeping fit to prevent obesity can be a fundamental part of preventing some diseases, such as type 2 diabetes. Smoking is related to many cancers, such as lung cancer and bladder cancer, but the risk factors for other cancers are less clear. Infectious diseases in poor countries, for example, Mali in West Africa, can develop in other ways. Malaria is one infectious disease in Mali that is transmitted through a mosquito. It is difficult to prevent this disease. As a visitor, you can take a medicine short term to prevent developing it, but such short-term prevention doesn't help people who live there year round. Other ways to prevent malaria include water management and using nets over beds to keep the mosquitoes from biting humans. Other diseases, such as guinea worm disease, can be prevented without any medical intervention at all. It requires community investment in keeping water sources clear of the disease.

Prevention is a fundamental part of community health. It requires a community of people to work together in prevention efforts, which may take many forms. In the "Social Ties" section, we learned through "Dadi's Chart" that family intervention in diabetes management can help people maintain healthy lives. Families and community efforts also can be very important in preventing disease. This might include encouraging people to get outside and exercise to prevent chronic diseases or encouraging people to work together to clean up water and other sanitation systems that foster infectious ones. This is a problem in many poor areas of low-income countries, such as Bangladesh, where there aren't organized sanitation systems, and diseases such as trachoma, which is carried by flies from human or animal waste to humans' eyes, become very problematic. Prevention means working together to do things that will improve individual health and the health of the community.

This section describes the ways in which prevention can impact people's lives by making sure they stay healthy and do not acquire the diseases common to the environments in which they live. "Gone Goes the Worm" demonstrates how Anok works to eliminate guinea worm disease by preventing people from spreading the disease through contaminated water sources. "A Pandemic Pig Tale" highlights another disease known as swine flu (or H1N1) that can be prevented by washing one's hands and covering one's mouth when coughing; the main intervention is education. "Route 100" highlights how a car accident associated with drunk driving not only causes personal injury but also can be a very traumatic experience. Finally, "Girl Parts" describes how cervical cancer can be easily prevented by routine screening.

As you read through this section, consider the following questions:

- What are some prevention efforts you have observed or taken part in your town or city? Can you think of ways a prevention effort for community health has influenced your health? Or has a disease been prevented for one of your family members?

- Think about the ways prevention might work differently in communities unlike your own. How might the environment in which people live influence how diseases develop?

- How are prevention efforts for communicable and noncommunicable diseases different? Are there similarities between what it takes to prevent these types of diseases?

19

Gone Goes the Worm

Adam Koon

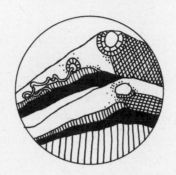

"Gone Goes the Worm" introduces Anok, who comes from a village in South Sudan, where guinea worm still remains a problem. Guinea worm is a disease that largely has been eliminated from the world as a result of the great efforts by the Carter Center based in Atlanta, Georgia. However, guinea worm still affects people in some of the most remote places on earth, such as villages in South Sudan. This story illustrates, through Anok's experiences as a village volunteer and then field officer for the Carter Center's program, that prevention is the only way guinea worm transmission can be stopped. People must learn how to prevent spreading guinea worm larvae into water sources, such as ponds and lakes. If the larvae aren't spread into these water sources, the disease won't spread to others. This concept may seem simple, but it is difficult when people do not have filtered water and must collect water daily from ponds and lakes. Guinea worm is one of the only diseases that has nearly been eliminated from the earth and cannot be prevented by medications or vaccines. This story illustrates how primary prevention is a fundamental part of the guinea worm eradication program in these remote villages.

Anok lives in a village called Dor, a traditional African village where people from the Dinka tribe live. The village is very poor. For twenty-two years, South Sudan fought a civil war with its neighbors to the north. Now the Republic of South Sudan is the world's newest country. The village of Dor is near the center of the new country. The war is over, but there are still no schools, clinics, or shops near Anok's village. People in Dor just eat what they can grow and follow their cows as they graze.

Sometimes Anok eats fish in a small market by the Nile river, the world's longest river. To get there, he walks for about half a day. In South Sudan it gets very hot, so frequently he drinks from a pond or river along the way. Many people, like Anok, walk places in South Sudan because they don't have cars. There are no cars in Dor; the village is too poor. They also drink water from ponds and streams because there are no water faucets there.

Anok lives in a simple hut, called a *tukul*, with a grass roof, dirt floor, and stick walls. When it rains, the water comes inside his hut and wakes him up at night. Sometimes people in his family get stung by scorpions or bitten by snakes at night because there is nothing to keep them out. When there is no moon, it is very dark inside his family's hut because Anok's family is too poor to own a light. As you can see, the village of Dor is not an easy place to live.

Anok's father has three wives. His mother is the second wife. Anok is fifteen years old and has a small sister and brother. Because he is not the child of his father's first wife, he didn't get to go to school. The school is in a village far away, and it takes several days to get there. Still, when Anok was young, he tried to get other kids to show him the things they learned at school.

YEAR 1

When Anok became a teenager, he was responsible for looking after the family's cows. The cows are the most valuable thing the family owns, so it is a very important responsibility. Other boys and men from the village of Dor also would look after their cows, and together they moved around in camps so that the cows could graze on fresh grass. These cattle camps, or *wutich*, are sometimes very far from the village of Dor. Anok and the other men would move with most of what they own to a new place, where they would stay for about one week. Then, when the grass was all eaten, they would move to a new cattle camp. They walked very far, spending most of the day on their bare feet. When it was very hot, or the mosquitoes were very bad, some boys would walk with their cows in the morning or at night. Because they would get thirsty, the boys would drink from any of the ponds or streams they passed on the way. They would do this all year long. Sometimes they would have big parties, where they would sing, dance, and wrestle. Other times people from faraway cattle camps came with weapons and stole their cattle. Life in a cattle camp was never boring.

One day, shortly after the rains began, Anok was in a cattle camp by the river Kamoch when a boy arrived from Dor. He had a message from Anok's mother. The messenger told Anok that his father's vision had gotten worse and that his sister had several *theiu*, or guinea worms. His mother needed him to come home to help with the garden and the goats.

Anok discussed the issue with one of his uncles and half brothers in the cattle camp. They agreed to look after Anok's cows while he helped his mother at home. Anok walked for six hours through a swamp to reach his home. When he got there, it was dark and his mother was bathing his little brother. She was happy to see him and squeezed his face and told him that he was getting fat in cattle camp. She pointed to his sister, lying on a thin reed mat on the ground. His sister groaned and told Anok that the theiu were very hot and burning. She pointed to two blisters about the size of a thumb on her left leg and three on her right. Anok didn't say anything, but he felt sorry for his little sister. He remembered how much he hated theiu when he was younger. He used to get them all the time, but it had now been a couple of years since his last worm. Many people in cattle camp got them too, but so far he had been lucky.

The next day, Anok rose early to help his mother in the garden while it was still cool. Then he went to find another boy to help the family with the goats. He went to the nearest neighbor's tukul, but there were no small children living there. He went to the next tukul and found a small boy, also sick with guinea worm. He could see the small blisters and the tiny white tips of the emerging worms. He went to five more families and all of them refused to help. He saw many young boys with guinea worm, and their families all were in the same situation as Anok's mother.

Anok grew frustrated and got into an argument with the woman of the last house. He asked why the boy there couldn't just look after a few extra goats. She got angry and told Anok that the boy doesn't even do a good job looking after his own family's goats. He spends too much time swimming and playing with his friends instead of taking care of his duties to the family. She refused to be responsible for her lazy boy losing another family's goats. She said that this was sure to create problems for her later.

Anok put his head down and returned home. He told his mother, who nodded. She didn't tell him that she had already asked all of her neighbors for help.

Then Anok reluctantly swatted at the behinds of the goats and took them out to feed. He took them far past the village's drinking ponds, where other children take their goats to feed. Once he was there, he saw some boys drinking from ponds and playing games with sticks. He went a different way to avoid being seen. He was embarrassed about having to do his sister's job. Looking after goats was for children. At fifteen, he was a man now and supposed to look after cows. He found a nice shady spot under a chum tree and hid out there while the goats picked at the leaves of nearby shrubs. This was how he spent several days while his sister was at home writhing in agony.

Then one day, just as he was about to leave with the goats, two men came to Anok's tukul. His mother was at a wedding for a relative in a village far away, so he greeted them. One of the men was his neighbor Kulang and the other was a man named Ngong from a different village by the river. They explained that Kulang was a village volunteer and his boss was Ngong, a field officer. Their jobs were to hunt guinea worms. They showed Anok a picture of a guinea worm and asked if he had seen any. Anok nodded and asked his sister to come out of the hut. After a few minutes, she shuffled up to the men, wiping away a tear.

Kulang, the village volunteer, asked her to sit down while he inspected her wounds. He then told Anok that he was going to start treating her. Anok was very interested. He didn't know that there was a correct way to treat guinea worm. He stood next to the field officer and watched as Kulang soaped down and cleaned his sister's legs. Then the volunteer soaked cotton gauze in water and placed them on his sister's blisters.

While Kulang was busy digging through his small medical kit for supplies, Ngong, the boss, started asking Anok questions. He asked him if he had just come from cattle camp and how long he planned on being home. He asked how the grass was in Kamoch and if there was any fighting in the area. Anok answered Ngong's questions while watching Kulang preparing his supplies. Ngong then asked Anok if he had seen anyone in cattle camp or in the village with guinea worm. Anok smiled and told him about his neighbors, and Ngong wrote down their names.

Anok laughed and asked him why he cared so much about this worm. Ngong pointed down to Anok's sister and said, "Your answer is there."

Anok's sister cried out in pain and beat the ground with her fist as Kulang squeezed puss from one of the blisters. He explained that often when people get guinea worm they also get infections. A tear started to roll down Anok's sister's cheek and she bit her bottom lip. More puss was coming out, with little streaks of blood in the yellow fluid. Kulang drizzled some water over the open wound and Anok leaned in closer. The village volunteer began to massage around the blister and Anok's sister grunted in pain.

As he worked closer to the wound, Anok began to see the worm. "It's there," said Kulang. The long tip emerged and with each squeeze it began to get longer. Pretty soon the spaghetti-like worm was about an inch long and curled slightly over the wound.

Kulang then stopped squeezing and started cleaning the wound with an orange soapy liquid. Then he cut a piece of gauze pad in half. Next he cut a little slit into it and tucked the worm through the slit. He pinched the worm and rolled the gauze pad.

Anok had never seen guinea worm treated like this. Kulang rolled the pad about one and half times around before it looked like the worm would snap. Then he let go of it and began massaging above the wound again. The girl grunted and hissed with pain. Her eyes now filled with tears.

Then Kulang picked up the rolled gauze with the worm and began to pull ever so slightly from side to side. Slowly, Anok could tell that more worm was coming out. The fresh part of the worm was wet, thick, and white. Kulang was able to rotate the cotton with the worm in it about three or four more times before the worm grew tight again. Then he left the roll pinned to the wound, grabbed another gauze pad, and bandage and began dressing the wound. He wrapped the bandage around her leg and over the wound several times until it was thick and secure. Then he tied it off and cut the excess bandage. It looked nice, and Anok was impressed.

Then he heard Ngong's voice behind him. "And that is how we treat guinea worm, my friend."

Kulang looked up at Anok from his perch above the girl's leg. Anok could see that the village volunteer was proud, and he thanked him. Kulang grew confused and said, "Oh, friend, we have only just started. I have to do the same thing to the other four blisters on your sister's legs." Anok laughed nervously and looked over at his sister, whose face was wet with tears.

Anok stayed and watched over Kulang's shoulder as the volunteer continued to work on his sister. In the meantime, Ngong began to ask the girl some questions.

"Where do you fetch water for the family?" he asked.

"We always use the *donghi* [hand pump], which is near our tukul," she replied.

Ngong nodded, looked at his clipboard, and asked, "But where do you go when the pump is broken?"

She shrugged and said, "I go to one of the small ponds nearby."

Ngong pressed her for more information. She then told him the names of the ponds and where they were located. The field officer then asked, "Do you use a *dhim* [filter] when you go to those ponds?"

She nodded, looked around shyly, and said, "I usually use a filter." Ngong didn't stop there.

"Where do you keep it?" he asked. She pointed to the rack made of sticks next to the smoldering fire. Ngong went over and pulled a brown cloth sack from underneath two of the sticks. "Is this it?" he asked, showing her the sack stuffed with *tompyn* (peanuts). She nodded, looking annoyed. Ngong then emptied the nuts onto the ground and showed the small sack to Anok.

"You see? Your mother has stitched the cloth filter into a bag to store things. You need to tell her that these filters are just to be used for filtering water. We're going to have to take this one with us. Kulang will give you a new one filter when we are finished."

Then Ngong noticed that the jerry can the family used to store water had brown water in it. He said to the girl, "I thought you go to the hand pump for water."

Wincing with pain as Kulang started to massage another part of her infected leg, she said, "I normally do, but now that I have guinea worm, my mother is the one to collect water. She is too busy with other things, so she doesn't have time to walk to the hand pump. Instead she just collects water from the nearest pond."

"And which pond is that?" Ngong asked.

"Angol," she replied, moving her head to show the pond's general direction.

Ngong wrote down the name of the pool and nodded to Kulang, who was now pulling on the girl's third worm.

"Did you hear that, Kulang?" Ngong asked. Kulang knew that it was his job to make sure that this kind of situation didn't happen. So instead of answering Ngong, he mumbled unhappily without looking up.

Anok asked Ngong a few questions as Kulang finished his work. Ngong looked up at the sky distractedly and began to hurry Kulang along. Before leaving he turned to Anok and said, "It sounds like this village is in bad shape. Maybe this village volunteer is tired and not doing his work. We're going to have a community meeting tomorrow about guinea worm. We need to work together to solve this problem. Please come tomorrow and we will answer all of your questions then."

"I will be there. Thank you," Anok said. He watched as they marched off through the high stalks of sorghum to his neighbor's hut.

YEAR 2

At that meeting a year ago, the community selected Anok to replace Kulang as village volunteer. Anok and Ngong now would work together at least twice a week. They would make maps of the villages and regularly hold community meetings. Even during the dry season, when there was no guinea worm, Anok would do his job of village volunteer. He would wake early every morning and walk to each tukul and chat with people there. He asked if they had seen guinea worm.

Then he would ask them, "Where are you getting your drinking water?" He knew everyone in the village already, but as a volunteer he had an excuse to talk with them more.

Even more important, he was their protector from guinea worm. He knew some of the village volunteers in other villages. They were lazy and didn't always do their jobs. Anok didn't care. Though he didn't get paid, he worked hard. He was proud of his job and wanted to prove it to his boss, Ngong. He did everything a village volunteer was supposed to do. Then he would ask to do more.

As a village volunteer, Anok was responsible for making sure that people knew about guinea worm, how to filter water, and what to do if they saw a worm. Anok also treated people with guinea worm and helped Ngong put a chemical in the water of drinking ponds. Once a month, Ngong organized a meeting with Anok and village volunteers from neighboring villages. They reviewed the proper steps for filtering water, treating guinea worm, and teaching people about the disease.

Ngong's boss, a Dinka man from a tribe on the other side of the river, also came to these monthly volunteer meetings. Anok knew this man, but he was very busy and rarely had time to spend with Anok. The man had fled war in his village when he was a boy, had grown up in Kenya, and then went to school in the United States. He now was here to help the people of Dor and several other villages. He was a great man and very well respected in the village. Anok followed Ngong's example and tried to always look very busy when this man was around.

One day, just as the rainy season began, an old man showed up as Anok was teaching a group of small children about guinea worm. Anok was using pictures from a special cloth flip chart to tell the story of guinea worm. The man walked through the group of children and asked, "What is this? Who are you?"

Anok recognized his uncle and laughed. He told him his father's name. The man still did not recognize Anok, but he nodded anyway.

"I am the village volunteer for guinea worm. Would you like to hear the story of guinea worm?"

"I already know all about guinea worm," said his uncle. "But I would like to see what the cloth flip chart has to say."

Anok then started from the beginning.

He showed the children and the old man each picture and asked them what they saw. In this way, Anok got them to tell the story of guinea worm. This way, they would remember it better.

Then after they were done, he reviewed the story. "First, a person with guinea worm enters the water. If nobody with guinea worm entered the water, then there would be no guinea worm the following year. It needs people to survive. Second, when the guinea worm is in the water, it releases its eggs. Third, somebody comes to drink the water with the eggs in it. Since the eggs are too small to see, the person doesn't know that they are in the water. If people use filters, then they will protect themselves from the eggs. If people don't use filters, then they might drink the eggs in the water. If they are filling jerry cans with water for their families and they don't use filters, then the eggs might get inside the jerry can. Fourth, if a person drinks the eggs, one year later a guinea worm will come out somewhere on his or her body. At this point, it is important for somebody to go fetch the village volunteer to help."

When the story was finished, the old man called out to Anok. "Young man, your story does not make sense to me. I see that guinea worm lives in the water, but how is it that some people get it and some people do not?"

Anok thought about this for a second and asked the man to explain further.

"I know you are young and you work hard, but I have trouble with this story," the man said. "Why is it that when the rains come my wife might get guinea worm, but I will not? Why might my boy get it, but the girl no. If it is in the water we drink, and we all drink the same water, then surely we should all get guinea worm? This is the problem I have with your story that it lives in the water. You tell us to believe you, but you cannot see these eggs. My wife drinks water and I drink water and only one of us gets guinea worm. This cannot be."

Anok thought carefully about this problem. Then he said, "Maybe you do not always drink the same water."

"Sure we do," the man replied. "There are two ponds by our house that we drink from. There is also a hand pump, but it does not work. My wife uses the same water for cooking and cleaning. We all use that water."

Without thinking, Anok then asked the man, "But is your wife always with you?"

The man's eyes widened, he stuck out his chest, and looked as if he was getting ready to strike Anok. "What are you saying, boy?"

Anok realized his error and tried to clarify. "What I mean is that sometimes we drink water from different places. Like you, for example. When you visit a cattle camp or travel to Pap to visit relatives, do you not drink water while you are away? I am sure your wife doesn't leave the home as she is a good mother, but is it possible that she has eaten with neighbors who have different water in their jerry cans? Have you not traveled to a river to collect fish and taken a drink while you were there? A year is a very long time for the guinea worm to grow in our bodies, which is why it is difficult for us to know which pond it came from."

When Anok finished, the man gazed off into the distance and quietly nodded. Anok put his flip chart into his medical kit and quickly moved away to the next tukul.

Later that day, when Anok was returning home, he found the first case of guinea worm for the year. His neighbor's son had a large blister on his ankle and it was causing him a lot of pain. The boy was about the same age as Anok's sister, and he often saw the two playing together. He went through all of the steps, but he did not see a worm that day.

Anok returned twice a day for four days before he finally saw the tip of the worm. He squeezed and massaged and did everything he was supposed to do, but the worm wouldn't come. After about a month of visiting every day, he finally removed the worm completely.

A full-length guinea worm can measure from the tip of your finger to your elbow. Some worms, like the one in his neighbor's son, can be very stubborn and take a long time to come out. But Anok didn't mind. Instead, he was more worried about a trend that he was noticing. Ngong and Anok were missing something.

A few weeks later, when there were about ten different people in the village with guinea worms, Anok decided to raise the issue with Ngong. What Anok wanted to do was to prevent people from getting guinea worm. First, though, he needed to find out where all these people were getting their worms. He had a hunch. He spoke with Ngong, and together they formed a plan.

YEAR 3

Another year passed, during which Anok became the field officer of Dor. Ngong was promoted to be the program officer in another area. For the first time in his life, Anok was getting paid to do a job. If he was lucky and nobody in his family got sick, he might be able to save enough money to buy cows for marriage. This would be very important because the life of a Dinka man remains incomplete until he has a wife and children. The more children (and wives), the wealthier the man.

Anok's new role required him to visit village volunteers and to make sure they were protecting the community from guinea worm. He visited new parts of the village and talked with more people. Most important, he frequently organized the community to solve problems. Together they were excited for this year. He reminded people that it would only take one person with guinea worm to enter the water for the whole community to be reinfected. If people refused to use filters or follow the community's rules, everybody could get guinea worm. Anok was confident that this would be the first year Dor was free of guinea worm.

The rains came late that year. Anok and the village volunteers spent a lot of time looking for cases of guinea worm. They looked and looked, but there was nothing to be found.

Halfway through the rainy season, Anok called the community together and asked if anyone had seen guinea worm. Nobody had. They reviewed the rules the community had made the previous year and they practiced filtering. They discussed other problems as well. The village volunteers were not active but wanted to be paid. Somebody drank water from a pond after the chemical was applied and said it tasted bad. A woman fetched water without a filter and was refusing to pay the fine of one chicken to the community committee. Somebody noticed that the children refused to wear their pipe filters when they left the village. Anok was tired, but he helped the community find solutions to each of these problems.

The rains came and went. Several cattle camps passed through Dor. Because there was no more grass, some people were moving to the river for the dry season. The color drained from Dor. Everywhere it was brown. Trees emptied and became dry. The thick carpet of trimmed grass turned to sand. And there was still no guinea worm to be found.

Anok was worried because many of the village volunteers were getting tired of having to look without finding any guinea worm. Sometimes they found a person with an infected wound, but no worm. Anok was convinced that they must be missing many people with guinea worm. He moved quickly from house to house, but by now they were sick of seeing him. People knew what to say and some even suggested to him that maybe the worms had gone somewhere else.

At the end of the year, Anok called one more community meeting. He announced that there had been no guinea worm that year but that they still must look hard. They must all keep practicing the things they learned about preventing guinea worm. The community began to complain and argue over things, and the noise grew louder. People started talking over one another.

Suddenly a small voice came from the back. People turned around and an old man approached the front. Everyone was silent. "I told you once that I did not believe in your story of guinea worm coming from the water," Anok's uncle said. "I told you that it made no sense for one person to be infected but another not. But you have showed me that it *is* that way. That this is how the worm works. I am not telling you this to say that an old man is foolish, but that we, the community, are right. We have been listening to this young boy, the volunteers, and the one they call Ngong. We have done what they said. We have learned how guinea worm lives. We have learned how to use filters. We have pulled together to make sure that we are stronger than our weakest members. We have showed what we can do as a community. So we should be happy."

The old man looked around at the empty faces. The volunteers and Anok stood at firm attention, their chests swollen with pride.

The man gazed off and asked simply, "So what next?"

Postscript: Though this story is a work of fiction, it was inspired by real events. The last case of guinea worm to be reported in the community of Dor was in September 2011. As of 2013, transmission of guinea worm disease is believed to have been eliminated in Awerial County, South Sudan. Gabriel Ngong, the program officer, has been moved to one of the last remaining strongholds of the disease in Warrap state. Anok Wol, the field officer, continues to fight guinea worm, and his wife recently gave birth to their first child.

20
A Pandemic Pig Tale

Erica Gibson

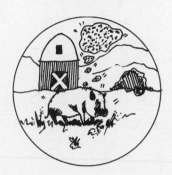

"A Pandemic Pig Tale" describes how a group of women respond to information about swine flu, also known as H1N1. H1N1, a newly identified virus, causes flu-type symptoms, but the illness is more severe and more deadly than the traditional flu. Peopled feared this new disease and held many different beliefs about where it came from and how it was transmitted. Soon after swine flu was discovered, scientists worked very hard to make a vaccine to prevent it. This story shows how Mayra's keen listening skills in school were important in educating her mother and other women in the village about the swine flu. H1N1 provides an excellent example of prevention, not only because there are clear avenues for preventing transmission of the disease but also because vaccinations, once they are developed, can prevent infection, even if someone is exposed to the flu. However, there are new types of flu every year, so scientists must continue to work hard to help protect community health.

A group of women sat around the table in Señora Garcia's kitchen making small talk while preparing tamales for the local celebration of Día de las Madres. Mother's Day, always held on May 10 in Mexico, was great cause for celebration. But this year, there was an atmosphere of trepidation in the small pueblo of Los Cielos due to the recent outbreak of *gripe porcina* (swine flu) in the area. People began coming down with flu-like symptoms—fevers, body aches, tiredness, and coughs—in early March, and after several died, samples were sent to the national lab to find out what was causing the illness. Some of the locals had their own explanations, even after hearing that the new disease was a form of influenza.

"We better enjoy this celebration since it's the last time we may come together as a community before someone figures out how to take care of this swine flu problem!" exclaimed Señora Garcia as she prepared the fillings for the tamales.

Señora Aguilar chimed in while chopping up cilantro. "I hear of more people each day who are getting sick from this new disease. That pig farm is the problem. With all of those stinking *malos aires* [bad air], it's no wonder people are dying."

All of the women nodded their heads in agreement. They had heard similar rumors about how swine flu had started at the industrial pig farm that was less than twenty kilometers from their village. Who could blame them for thinking that this operation was the cause of yet another hardship? The odors from the industrial farm were brought on the winds, and the stench produced by thousands of pigs living in crowded conditions would sometimes settle over the town. Rumors were circulating that the odors and the miasma, or bad air, was the cause of people falling ill. Even before this outbreak, the industrial farm had had a large impact on the local area and played a role in dividing families.

Most of the men in the village had immigrated to the capital or to the United States in search of work because the local areas that were once farmed as a cooperative had been taken over by large-scale industrial farming organizations like the pig farm. These industrial farms were built by outside nations in a push to buy up cheap land. They would bring in their own workers and employ very few locals, putting the majority of the men in the area out of work. The men were forced to travel farther and farther away from their homes to find work. Once they gained employment, the men sent money home to their families to support the household, but they were not there to help with the day-to-day problems women faced in caring for their families. The men had left Los Cielos a village of women, children, and the elderly—the people left included two of the groups most affected by swine flu: children under five years old and adults age sixty-five and older.

Mayra and Rosa helped their mother, Señora Garcia, prepare the hojas (cornhusks) for the addition of the masa (cornmeal) and fillings. The girls began helping their mother with many of the cooking and cleaning chores when their father left to find work in the capital. Although this was work that women would commonly do in their community, their mother also had to take on many other responsibilities, making it difficult to take care of daily chores on her own. While cleaning and soaking the hojas, Mayra's ears perked up as she heard her mother speak. "Did you hear the school will be closed for the entire week of Mother's Day?"

The other women nodded, acknowledging that they too had heard that the school would be closed. Their solemn responses indicated that it was not, however, a cause for celebration. Mayra attempted to hide her smile, as she was excited to be home from school, but she knew that an outbreak of gripe porcina was not cause for celebration.

"The school officials say that they must close the school and public offices by order of the government to try to prevent this gripe porcina from spreading any further," their mother continued. "We're lucky that our village has not been affected as badly as some of the other areas nearby. This sickness is spreading fast."

"I heard the pigs were the first to get the sickness at the giant factory pig farm down the road," said Señora Cuevas. "How can a pig disease make people sick? What are we supposed to do to prevent this disease from making us and our children sick?"

"Well, for one, we're not going to be eating any pork in our tamales this year!" responded Mayra's mother. "I don't want to get sick from eating a diseased pig."

"Mama, you can't get the flu from eating pork!" exclaimed Mayra. "Our teacher, Señor Lima, told us that swine flu is just like any other flu.

It spreads through the air, not through the meat of pigs." Señora Garcia gave Mayra a stern look and said, "Well maybe it is all the bad air floating around from the pig farm. How does your teacher know this? Is he a doctor too?"

"No, Mama, but we read an article in the newspaper about swine flu and how it is passed by germs from one person to another. It's not the air itself that is bad, just the bad germs floating in the air. Señor Lima told us we had to be careful and cover our mouth when we sneeze or cough because this is how germs are spread. We also have to be sure to wash our hands."

Señora Garcia wasn't convinced by Mayra's statement. "How do we know that he is right? We need to talk to a health worker. I wonder if doña Alma is available to tell us about this illness. She is always trying to convene the women into one place, and since we are all here making tamales together, maybe we should ask her to come speak to us. I could think of no one better to educate us than the *promotora* [health promoter]."

Mayra and Rosa nodded in agreement.

"Mijas, why don't you run together to the health clinic to ask doña Alma if she might have time to speak with us after she finishes seeing people at the clinic?"

"Yes, Mama!" the girls answered in unison. Rosa ran out of the hot kitchen first, trying to beat her older sister to the health clinic.

Doña Alma was having a busy day in the health clinic. She was both the public health nurse and promotora for the village. As the only medical provider in the village, she had multiple jobs: she gave educational talks (*platicas*), which were conversations with the villagers about how to stay safe and healthy, and served as the main health provider in the clinic. Her two roles of educator and caregiver made her schedule very busy.

That day the clinic was open for vaccination day, and mothers brought their babies for checkups and vaccines. A vaccine is a medicine that is given to people before they get sick to prevent them from getting different illnesses. The body is protected from getting sick in the future because the body makes antibodies as a response to the vaccine. These antibodies know exactly how to fight the virus if the body is exposed to it in the future. Each mother is responsible for making sure her child's vaccines are up to date and for remembering to bring her child's vaccination card to the clinic.

On the day that Mayra and Rosa arrived in the clinic, many women had asked doña Alma if there was a vaccine to protect themselves and their children against the new flu that was making people so ill. Because it was such a new disease, doña Alma was unable to provide the new mothers or their babies with vaccines to prevent swine flu.

Mayra and Rosa waited patiently to explain to doña Alma that their mother wanted her to come and speak with the *tamalada* (tamale party) to share information about swine flu with the group of assembled women. While they waited, Rosa called Mayra over to a giant poster hung on the wall of the clinic. Rosa was still too young to read, but she could see from the pictures on the poster that the painted faces represented people who were sick.

Rosa pointed out each picture and said, "Look Mayra! That person is coughing, that one looks hot, and that one has a headache."

Mayra read aloud from the poster. "These are symptoms of influenza: cough, runny nose, fever, and headache. If you have any of these symptoms you can receive free treatment at this health clinic."

Rosa asked Mayra, "What's 'fluenza' mean?"

"Influenza is the swine flu that the women were talking about," Mayra replied. "That's why we're here to see doña Alma. Hopefully she will have time to come talk to Mama and the other women about the swine flu this afternoon so Mama will see that I am right. I don't want her to be scared to use pork in the tamales because of the swine flu. Pork tamales are my favorite!" she added with a smile.

After some time, doña Alma finished vaccinations for the day and came to speak with Mayra and Rosa in the waiting room. The two girls took turns explaining that their mother asked them to invite doña Alma to speak with the women at the tamalada about where swine flu originated and how it was spread.

"Our Mama is worried that we could get sick from eating pork, but my teacher, Señor Lima, told us that swine flu is like regular flu and we have to be careful not to spread germs," explained Mayra.

"I'm glad you were paying attention in class, Mayra," said doña Alma as she smiled at the two girls. "Now, let's go see if we can help the women understand the swine flu."

Mayra and Rosa ran ahead to tell their mother and the other women that doña Alma was on her way to speak to the women about gripe porcina.

"Thank you, girls. Doña Alma will surely be able to sort this out. We can have a platica with her out in the courtyard while the tamales are steaming," said Señora Garcia as she wiped her apron.

All of the women wandered out of the hot, steamy kitchen into the shaded courtyard to greet doña Alma. Everyone in the village had great respect for doña Alma because she was so knowledgeable about health and worked tirelessly to make sure everyone remained healthy. This was not an easy task for the one trained health worker in the village. Doña Alma not only worked on vaccinations but also made sure that villagers had accurate knowledge about health and sanitation issues.

Doña Alma arrived to warm greetings from the women at the tamalada. Mayra's mother offered her a warm tea and they all sat down together. "So," said doña Alma in a kind, unthreatening tone, "what is this I hear about you not wanting to make pork tamales, Señora Garcia?"

"This new disease is called swine flu, right?" said Señora Garcia. "And I have heard lots of rumors that it started in the industrial pig farms outside of town and that the disease passed to people because they were eating the meat of sick pigs. But others have said it's the bad air that blows in from the pig farm that is causing so much sickness. I just don't know what to think anymore, but I want to keep my family safe. I think it's better to stay away from the pigs altogether rather than take a chance when I don't know how this new disease is transmitted."

"I understand, Señora Garcia, and you are right to be concerned. I will help clear up these misunderstandings," replied doña Alma. "Now, who else has heard rumors about swine flu?"

"I heard that the poor pregnant woman who died in the village down the road had eaten pork that her husband brought home from the farm," said Señora Cuevas. "Now he is all alone raising their two-year-old son!"

Many of the other women chimed in, saying, "Yes, I heard that too!"

"Did a pregnant woman really die from swine flu, doña Alma?" asked Mayra.

"Yes, child. She was just a few months pregnant when she became sick. This was just as the new disease was starting to spread. Her symptoms appeared to be the same as the regular flu we see here during the winter months, but it was already springtime and no one had been sick from the flu for more than a month. She was coughing and had a runny nose and fever, and she complained of aches and pains. The doctor didn't know that there was a new type of flu and so he told her to go home and rest. Unfortunately, her body could not fight off the sickness and she died. Now we know that this may be swine flu, and we can start to give medicine as soon as we know that a person is sick."

"Was it because she ate pork from a pig that had been sick?" Señora Garcia inquired, turning her head and tweaking her ear toward doña Alma so as not to miss a beat.

"How many of you believe that you can get swine flu from eating pork from a sick pig?" Doña Alma asked the group. Each woman raised her hand, with the exception of Mayra and Rosa. Nodding at the two girls, doña Alma continued. "And Mayra, what do you believe?"

"Well, Señor Lima told us that we can only become sick from swine flu if we get germs from someone else who is already sick."

"How can you get these germs?" the promotora asked with a supportive grin.

"If a sick person coughs and doesn't cover their mouth, or if they cough into their hand and then shake hands with you, the germs can pass to you. If you play with the same toys as a sick kid, then you can get the germs off of the toys too." Mayra was excited to share her knowledge with doña Alma, a very powerful leader in the village, and was pleased that doña Alma responded so positively to what she had learned in school.

"Very good! Mayra, you are absolutely right." Doña Alma paused for a minute and pivoted from Mayra to face the group of ladies whose faces still appeared unconvinced. "Can anyone tell me how to prevent the spread of these swine flu germs?"

"I can!" shouted Rosa as she jumped to her feet. "You have to cover your mouth when you cough, and you have to wash your hands before you eat, and after you have been playing outside or with other kids."

"That is a great start, Rosa, and remember you have to use soap each time you wash your hands, and wash for fifteen to twenty seconds or the germs won't die." Doña Alma continued, facing the women, "Now, what about eating pork? Can this make you sick with swine flu?"

"No, ma'am!" Mayra and Rosa shouted in unison.

"The girls are right," said doña Alma with a serious face. "Eating pork will not give you swine flu. You can't get swine flu from eating cooked pork, even if the pig that the pork came from was sick. Swine flu is like the other kind of flu. It is a contagious virus that is spread through coughing, sneezing, or coming into contact with the germs. The best way to avoid becoming sick is to stay away from people who are already sick. This is why they are closing the school and the government offices for the entire week. Many people in our area have become sick and it's only a matter of time before swine flu spreads throughout our village."

"So the germs can be spread through the air?" asked Señora Aguilar, the wife of a government officer. "It's just as I thought, *bad air*! All of that horrible smell from those pigs!"

"But Señora Aguilar, it's not the bad smell that spreads the disease," said Mayra. "Nobody in our village is sick yet, and we have to smell that every time the wind blows east!"

Doña Alma continued. "Yes, the germs are passed through the air but only from people who are sick with the virus, not from the odor."

The women murmured in agreement as the village had been dealing with the smell for many months before anyone became sick. One of the shy, younger women raised her hand to ask doña Alma a question. "So if it's the germs that make people sick, like Mayra said, why is this disease called swine flu? Did it come from pigs originally?"

"It was likely passed from pigs to humans at some point, which is why it is called 'swine flu,' but the scientific name is H1N1," responded doña Alma. "It may have been transferred from pigs to humans locally, but it also may have been brought to our area from one of the men returning from the capital or from the United States. Increased migration back and forth between areas with different illnesses is causing germs to spread faster than previously possible." Doña Alma went on to explain that the tiny pueblo of Los Cielitos was once isolated from the spread of many diseases, but with increasing globalization, such as the industrial pig farm that moved in and the flow of men in and out of the area looking for work, new pathways for germs to spread have opened up.

"But how do you know if someone has the swine flu?" asked Señora Aguilar. "My uncle has been coughing and sneezing for days! Does he just have a cold or does he have H1N1?"

"It sounds like your uncle may just have a cold or allergies at this time of year," responded doña Alma. "The symptoms for swine flu are just like other types of flu. If you start coughing, have a runny nose, sore throat, headache, body ache, and chills, you may have swine flu. Unfortunately, the test for distinguishing swine flu from other types of flu is only available in certain laboratories in the capital for now. We can't know for sure whether someone has this particular type of flu, but we can give medication to try to help people with flu symptoms get better faster. We can also take precautions to prevent the spread of the flu. One of the ways to prevent the spread of germs that can make you sick is to keep your house clean. You can mix a solution of one part bleach to four parts water to disinfect areas where germs may be spread such as countertops, plastic toys, door handles, and bathrooms."

"How easy is it for swine flu to spread to other people?" Mayra's mother inquired. "Should we stay away from Señora Aguilar since she has been by her uncle who's sick?"

"As long as Señora Aguilar didn't get too close to her uncle, and she washed her hands after she left his house, everything should be fine. But swine flu is contagious for up to seven days. In the wintertime the government sends us special vaccines to help prevent the flu, but there are no vaccines available to prevent swine flu yet. The only way to avoid getting sick right now is to stay away from people who you know are sick and to keep your houses and your families as clean and germfree as possible." As doña Alma got up to leave, she said, "I hope I have been able to answer some of your questions about swine flu."

As the women thanked doña Alma for the information, the timer buzzed in the kitchen indicating that the tamales were ready to be removed from the steamer. Señora Garcia called Mayra to help her in the kitchen while the other women continued chatting.

"Mayra, I am so proud of you," her mother said as she placed her hand on Mayra's head. "You are paying attention in class and learning so much. You are able to teach your younger sister Rosa and I the things that you have learned to help keep our family healthy and safe. Thank you, mija."

"You're welcome, Mami!" exclaimed Mayra as she hugged her mother. "Now that we know it is safe, could we please make some pork tamales?"

"Absolutely," her mother said with a wide grin. "But first take doña Alma some of these tamales that are already prepared to thank her for coming to speak with us today."

21

Route 100

Suzanne Farrell Smith

"Route 100" follows the path of Shannon, a ten-year-old girl who witnessed a car crash that killed a woman and left behind her three daughters. The twenty-one-year-old driver who caused the accident had been drinking and walked away with minor injuries. Years later, when Shannon turns fifteen, she refuses to start driver's education, even though she is of age in her home state of Vermont. Vermont is among those states with the highest percentage of teens driving under the influence of alcohol or illicit drugs. Fortunately, due to efforts by local governments, law enforcement, schools, and private organizations, drunk and drugged driving is a decreasing problem across the United States. But driving under the influence of alcohol or drugs remains a leading cause of preventable death by injury in this country. It is important for young people to understand the physical dangers of driving under the influence as well as the legal and psychological consequences.

Shannon stared at her father, searching his face for a sign that he was joking. After all, he couldn't be serious about *this*. She watched his mouth open and close. But she stopped understanding his words after the first few.

"It's time for you to learn how to drive," he said.

Didn't he remember her terror? Didn't he know about the nightmares? The panic attacks? The envelope stuffed with yellowed newspaper clippings, collected from that time, five years ago?

"Here's the plan," her mother had said that morning, as they ate buckwheat pancakes. "As soon as breakfast is over, get upstairs and pack a backpack. Don't forget a book for bedtime. And Lulu. I'll bring some snacks for us. Dad, grab the camera and make sure the batteries are charged!"

Shannon was ten. So was Lulu the stuffed elephant, Shannon's constant companion since she was a baby.

"Careful, sweets," said Shannon's mother. "You're going to make yourself sick." Shannon was wolfing down her pancakes.

"I can't wait!" Shannon said, after swallowing the last bite. She bounded upstairs to pack her bag.

Shannon and her parents were heading to Montpelier for the annual Fourth of July parade and fireworks. The capitol of Vermont, Montpelier was a small city. But to Shannon, whose tiny town had about five hundred residents and a single main street through the village center, Montpelier seemed huge. All across the United States people celebrated the country's independence, and Montpelier always put on a great show.

She'd grown up knowing nothing but rural life: the bindweed, daisies, ferns, clover, and irises in the fields near her house; the gentle slopes of the valley leading into the Green Mountains; the bees, butterflies, dragonflies, and moths that called the woods home. She knew the trees too. Maple and walnut, oak and ash. And endless numbers of pine trees.

Every year, though, Shannon left her natural paradise and climbed into the station wagon for the three-and-a-half-hour drive along Route 100 to Montpelier. They could make the trip in two hours if they took the highway, but Shannon's family enjoyed sight-seeing along one of the nation's most picturesque roads. In fact, any time they went pretty much anywhere at all, they chose the narrow, winding roads. Such was life in a rural New England.

The drives, for Shannon, were always pleasant, and this year's ride to Montpelier was no exception. Shannon never read or listened to music in the car. She watched, instead, how the roadside scenery changed with each new bend, how the wildflowers leaned into thickets, how the trees sometimes clumped together and other times spread wide apart, how each mountain peak—pointed or rounded—came into view, grew larger, then disappeared behind her.

When they arrived in town, the parade was just gearing up. Shannon happily bounced up and down between her parents as the family watched a pickup truck carrying a band playing banjos and congas and even an Australian didgeridoo. The mayor, dressed as Uncle Sam, waved to the crowds in time with a barbershop quartet. A woman danced in a costume made entirely of buttons, a man balanced on a unicycle, a troop of children held banners proclaiming love and peace.

By the end of the day, after they'd trekked up the steep hill to the local college campus, stood watching the fireworks crackle and explode over town, and trekked down again to their hotel, Shannon's feet were sore. She pulled off her shoes and socks and rubbed them, absentmindedly thumbing thick calluses and the tender spot where she'd gotten a splinter some days before.

The next morning, Shannon and her parents piled back into the car for the long drive home. The day had dawned beautifully clear. Shannon played her favorite car game: counting the species of flowers and trees. Her father drove just under the speed limit, so Shannon had plenty of time to count.

Maple trees. Daisies. A wooden bridge stretching over a stream lined with beech trees.

Not too many cars were on the road this early. Route 100 was slightly damp with dew, and Shannon could see a faint set of tire tracks on the road ahead, like a wake. She glanced back to see if their car left a similar wake, and saw just one other car behind them, a silver minivan. A woman was driving. Shannon could tell she was a young woman but couldn't tell *how* young because the morning sun glinted off the windshield. Without knowing why, Shannon noticed that the woman was pretty.

In the distance, the mountain peaks met the sun and glistened green, while a white church spire stuck out among the lush green tree cover. Shannon's eyes grew heavy. As her parents chatted away in the front seat about a new garden project, Shannon let the rolling countryside send her into a Green Mountain trance.

Pine trees. Tall and elegant with straight, straight trunks.

Then, out of the blue, her mother yelled, "Watch out!"

The car swerved violently to the right, onto the shoulder of the road. Shannon was thrown into the door, hard. She righted herself and watched in horror as a small blue car barreled toward them on their side of the road. It didn't seem to be slowing down. Her father fought to keep their car under control and out of the path of the oncoming vehicle. The blue car streaked past them. Seconds later, a terrible noise overcame Shannon's ears and mind, the explosive sound of crunching metal and splintering glass.

Their car came to a stop some fifty yards beyond where they had first swerved. Shannon and her parents sat still for a moment, in shock, before Shannon's mom started to cry, her shoulders shaking. Her father reached out his hand and placed it on her mother's knee. "We're all right," he said, his voice even but hollow. "We're all right."

Shannon craned her neck to look back. The small blue car was stopped in the middle of the road. Something was odd. Where was the silver van?

She scanned the scene. That's when she saw it. But it didn't look like a van anymore; it looked like a small mountain of crushed metal, stuck among the beautiful trees, the pine trees they had just passed on the side of the road. Shannon stared. At first she thought about the van itself. She couldn't get her mind to understand how a car could go from looking like a silver box to a crushed, twisted mound, like a frightening version of the Green Mountains she loved.

"We need to get help," Shannon's father was saying, as her mother, still crying, pulled out her cell phone. Her father turned around and looked directly at Shannon.

"Don't move. Don't get out of the car, Shannon. Do you hear me?"

She nodded. But once her mother was on the call, reporting the accident, she had to get out of her tiny backseat. She disobeyed her father, slid quietly out of her seat belt, and got out, walking softly, quietly, back along the road's shoulder. From the side of the road, she could see a man in the blue car. He was pinned by his airbag. He was shaking his head side to side. The front of his car was completely smashed in. When Shannon looked more closely at the driver, she saw that he was very young.

Shannon's father was approaching the silver mess. Emergency vehicles seemed to take forever to arrive. Shannon's mother came to her and, thankfully, didn't admonish her for getting out. Instead, she gently put her arm around Shannon's shoulders and guided her back to their car. Shannon noticed the smell of pine was strong. For the first time in her life, it didn't smell fresh and comforting. Instead, the smell was overwhelming. Shannon felt suffocated.

Hours passed before they could leave. Shannon's parents both gave statements to the police and then they lingered, wanting to help in some way.

Back on the road, Shannon's father drove slowly. Shannon held Lulu tight. Everyone was quiet.

"Where was the other driver?" Shannon asked, breaking the silence.

"What?" her father replied.

"I saw the man in the blue car," Shannon said. "But I didn't see the pretty woman who was driving the silver van."

Both her parents were quiet. Then, finally, her father said, "Shannon, she was still in the car."

Shannon couldn't believe that. It had to be a mistake. No one could be inside that van. It had been completely crushed by the blue car, by all the trees that it struck, by the cold, wet, hard road.

No one was in that van. There had to be a mistake.

The next morning, Shannon and her parents looked in the newspaper for news of the accident. On page 3, they found it. Shannon wasn't ready to hear the headline. "Car Traveling in Wrong Direction Causes Fatal Accident."

"Dad," said Shannon. "Fatal. You mean, the man died?"

"No, honey. The man, it seems, is fine. He was barely hurt. He's twenty-one. The woman he hit, the woman who had been driving behind us, she died in the crash."

"But I don't understand."

"I know, honey. It's just awful." Shannon's mother got up for more coffee, stopping by her father's chair for a moment to rest her fingers lightly on his shoulders. The house felt cold, even though the hot July morning was pressing in on all sides.

After they had finished the paper, Shannon's mother threw it into the recycling bin and left the kitchen. Shannon approached the bin. She wanted that paper. She retrieved it and snuck it upstairs to her room. The next day, and the next, she learned more about the accident from the papers. The woman was a mother. Three daughters at home. Her husband and children were devastated by her death. A funeral was planned for Friday. The young man in the blue car had been driving—speeding, in fact—on the wrong side of the road. One witness to the accident, Shannon's father, had jerked his car out of the way. But the woman behind them hadn't seen the oncoming car in time. She was hit with the full force of the little blue car. She died instantly.

The driver of the blue car, Shannon learned, had been drinking all night, celebrating the Fourth of July. He had stayed at a friend's house and was still drunk when he got in his car to head home the following morning. Home was an hour away. Along Route 100.

Shannon kept all the papers. Three daughters. What were they going to do without their mom? As sad as she was for the family, Shannon couldn't help but feel lucky. It could have been her mom or dad that got killed. It could even have been her. But somehow she and her parents survived. They were still here, still eating pancakes with homemade syrup. The woman who died would never again make pancakes and syrup for her young children.

Shannon also felt guilty. If her family hadn't been driving in front of the woman, she might have seen the blue car coming. She might have gotten out of the way.

Mostly, Shannon wondered what would have happened if that man hadn't been drinking. He would have seen the road clearly. He would have driven the way her parents always drove. The pretty woman in the silver minivan would have returned home to her family. His choice, to get in his car and drive, ended a woman's life. It was too much for Shannon to understand.

"Mom, I want to go to the funeral."

"Shannon, it's very far away. They lived north of Montpelier. The woman was traveling down here to see her sister."

"Please, Mom, I want to go. I think we should."

In the end, Shannon's parents agreed. The day was unbearably hot and sunny, weird for a funeral, Shannon thought. In a daze, she watched the young husband weep, watched his daughters stand stone-faced next to the casket. How would they go on?

She continued to collect articles until there were no more. It was deemed manslaughter. The man had been drunk. He'd been up all night partying with his friends, and still had a high level of alcohol in his blood when he got in his car to drive home.

After the crash, Shannon stayed very close to home. Her feet became thick with calluses since, once school started again, she preferred to walk the mile there rather than catch a ride on the bus or with her parents. She didn't want them to drive either, and she became obsessed with the weekends when they could explore the woods or just sit in the yard, reading, enjoying the weather.

The nightmares started a few months later. Just when Shannon thought she was starting to feel better, she found herself in the same terrible nightmare over and over again.

She's walking in the middle of a road, trying to keep balance, one foot in front of the other along the double yellow line. She hears the faint hushing of wind through the pine trees when out of nowhere a bright-blue car comes speeding toward her, its headlights flashing. Shannon looks at the driver and sees herself behind the wheel, her own eyes wide and wild through the windshield.

Just before the car hit her, Shannon always woke up sweating and crying, unable to get back to sleep for fear of seeing herself driving the blue car again.

Mornings were torture. Because she wanted to walk to school, Shannon had to get up especially early, but she was so tired from not getting enough sleep. She didn't feel like breakfast most mornings, her stomach knotted up from the terror. By the time she got to school, she was so sleepy and hungry she couldn't concentrate in class. On her first report card of fifth grade, Shannon's teacher wrote, "Shannon seems distracted and has a difficult time staying focused." Shannon didn't feel that way; she liked school and wanted to learn, to please her teachers, and to have fun with her classmates. But she felt so tired all day, and so awake and scared all night. It was like the crash had flipped her life upside down.

Shannon forgot what it felt like to not be afraid, to climb a tree or launch herself from the tire swing into the swimming hole. And she was afraid that she would always be afraid, that she would never again be able to do the things she used to love.

Shannon's behavior didn't go unnoticed in her house. Her parents, so used to their upbeat, energetic ten-year-old daughter, wondered what to do for Shannon as she turned into a quiet, nervous eleven-year-old girl. Shannon didn't tell them about her nightmares, but she didn't have to. They knew that since the crash, Shannon had suffered. Still, they wanted to give their daughter as much time as she needed to settle her fears and recover her sense of wonder about the world.

But a year after the crash, when the Fourth of July approached and Shannon's parents asked her if she wanted to go, she said no. She was afraid of Route 100, afraid of what used to be the most beautiful stretch of road in all of Vermont, afraid of the trees that crushed the silver van. They stayed home.

"Shannon," said her mother the morning of the holiday, "Dad and I have been talking for a while about this, and we think it's time we got you some help."

"What does that mean?" asked Shannon. She didn't know anything about therapy. She only knew how scared she felt.

"We think you could use someone to talk to. Someone who isn't one of us."

"About the crash?" Shannon said, guessing her mother's reason.

"Yes. About the crash. And about how you feel now. The crash was a scary and sad event. But it happened a year ago. We think you need help to understand it and to not feel afraid of it anymore. We should have done this a long time ago."

It took many visits with the therapist, but Shannon grew less afraid. She learned how to talk about her nightmares. She learned about trauma, and that many people, adults and children alike, feel scared long after traumatic events are over. She learned to say to herself, *Just because something terrible happens doesn't mean it's going to happen again*. Mostly, she learned that she was still Shannon, that she still loved counting trees and being with her family and celebrating holidays like the Fourth of July, and that she could enjoy all those things again, even if it meant a long car trip.

Even though Shannon began to feel better, she thought every single day of that family, of those three girls, and eventually grew to see them in her mind as sisters. She ached to share with them her own loving mother, as if she could somehow help ease their pain.

Now, five years later, Shannon was fifteen, and her father wanted her to start taking driving lessons. "It's time for you to get your permit," he said. He handed her a pamphlet from a local driving school. "It's time for you to get out there, to explore a little bit." But Shannon wasn't listening anymore. She couldn't do it. She couldn't. All her old fears had come back. What if another drunk driver was on the long, winding, empty stretches of Vermont roads? It was one thing to be able to ride in the car with her parents again. She couldn't get behind the wheel of a car herself.

But those girls. Since the day of the funeral, Shannon had thought about visiting them, about making friends, writing them letters, bringing them presents. But they lived so far away. To see them, Shannon would have to be able to drive.

She took the pamphlet to her room and closed the door. For the first time in a long while, she pulled out the envelope full of articles about the crash. She read them and looked at the pictures. Now that she was fifteen, she wondered what happened to the man, the man who was hardly older than a teenager, only just legally allowed to drink, when he made his terrible choice. Did he ever get past it? Did he learn from it?

She looked at the driving-school pamphlet. On its front, a girl Shannon's age was sitting at the wheel of a car, holding a set of keys and smiling. "Learn to Drive," it read above the car in block letters. Underneath: "Be independent. Be responsible. Be safe."

I don't need to drive to be independent, Shannon thought. But she was curious. She opened to the first page and saw a list of the most common bad driving habits. Speeding, following too closely, not buckling up. Then number four: driving while impaired.

The next page showed a contract new drivers can sign with their families. Parents and teenagers alike pledge to drive safely. The pamphlet went on to name people and organizations working to make the roads safer: the government was writing stricter guidelines about driving while distracted or impaired, law enforcement was paying closer attention to what was happening on the road, community organizations like Mothers Against Drunk Driving were holding rallies and vigils to remind people to be safe, schools were including responsible driving in their curriculum, teens who had survived car crashes were traveling the country to tell their stories.

There was so much Shannon hadn't thought about. As she read, she learned that traffic crashes were the most common cause of injury and death in teenagers from fifteen to nineteen years old. She learned that distractions, like phones and music and talking with passengers, could be just as dangerous as drinking. Ideas started to form in Shannon's mind. She could start an awareness group in her school. She could ask a police officer to visit. When she grew older, she could mentor new drivers about safety.

Slowly, Shannon's fear hardened into resolve. She decided that she needed to get past her fear, once and for all. *Just because something terrible happens doesn't mean it's going to happen again.* She would learn to drive. She would drive carefully. She would treat driving as a critical responsibility. Shannon wouldn't only learn how to drive, she'd become a model driver. She couldn't hide from the road forever. Instead, she'd help make the road safer for herself, her family, and people like the pretty young mother of three.

The next day, as she signed up for the driver's education class, Shannon thought, This is not just for me. This is for my sisters.

22
Girl Parts

Judi Marcin

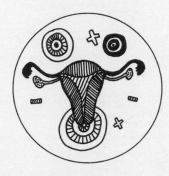

"Girl Parts" is the story of a teenage boy struggling with the possibility that his mother may have cervical cancer. Cervical cancer is one of the most common reproductive health problems, affecting women not only in the United States but also in other countries. It is the leading cause of cancer death among women in low-income countries because many people do not have access to cervical cancer screening. On the other hand, in the United States and other high-income countries, people with access to routine medical care receive Pap smears to screen for abnormal cells in the cervix. These abnormal cells are caused by a very common sexually transmitted infection (STI) called human papillomavirus (HPV). By identifying these abnormal cells early, many women receive treatment to prevent these abnormal cells from becoming cancer. However, women who are not regularly screened and develop advanced cases of cervical cancer are more likely to die from the disease. This story explores the relationship between a young man and his mother and how he comes to terms with his lack of understanding about the female body. It is a story of family and how life's stressors can bring out the strengths of individuals as well as the family

unit. Love, empathy, and communication are key components in the success of this mother-son relationship.

Mama came home and plopped her purse on the counter. She took off her Macy's name tag and set it in the windowsill in front of the kitchen sink. Jared didn't have to see her do this; he just knew. In the thirteen short years of his life he had come to know her well. It had been only the two of them for a long time and he had learned that she was predictable. A half-drunk cup of coffee down the drain before work, name tag on windowsill after work. Why not just pour yourself half a cup and save the dumping out? he wondered but never asked. Coffee in the morning, not at night, walking around in stocking feet most of the time, and looking at the paper but not reading it much. That was Mama, someone who never changed and seemed comfortable in her own routine. But routine or not, she had worked hard to make their life better. She had gotten a job as a clerk and was now manager of the housewares department at Macy's largest store in the city. Jared knew it hadn't been easy.

Papa left them when Jared was four or five. He might have been six. Neither of them ever talked about him much. Jared didn't remember a lot about his leaving. Papa had always been gone so much for work that his not being around, ever again, didn't seem like much of a change. But Jared learned, early on, how difficult it was for Mama. She would cry when least expected, sometimes at the breakfast table while he played with his Legos, sometimes in the car driving to the grocery store, sometimes in front of the TV when her favorite love story came on. And sometimes just looking at a jar of jelly would bring her to tears. As often as he could, Jared would sit down next to her, put his head in her lap, and tell her how much he loved her, and how even when he was grown he would stay with her always. Mama would brush the hair out of his eyes and smooth it down behind his ears. She would lovingly trace his eyebrows with her fingertip and Jared would drift off to sleep.

But that was then. For years, he had stopped putting his head down in her lap. He had long quit telling her every day that he loved her. Things that made sense and seemed so true when he was six or eight had become confusing at eleven, then twelve, then thirteen. He had changed, and so had his life and his priorities. Mama was no longer the center of his universe. School, friends, and his Xbox had won his heart, attention, and focus. For the first time, he started seeing a world outside of their two-bedroom brick house. Now, he realized, he wanted a life of his own someday, away from home. Guilt had settled in his chest; he had made so many promises that he'd never be able to keep. He knew someday he would move out and move on. Maybe he'd join the army or go to college. Maybe he'd travel, see the world, work enough here and there for food or a place to crash. His future seemed exciting. Mama's life was routine, dull.

But one day, as he was preparing to guide Admiral Zena and Commander Riggs through the alien lair, Jared heard the once-familiar sound of crying again. He stopped clicking the controller and paused the game. Without moving his eyes off the screen, he listened. Yep, he thought, crying. He tried to guess what might have triggered it. He wanted to keep playing but was concerned. This was his chance to help. Jared tried to refocus on the game, but he knew the right thing to do was to check on Mama.

"Mama, I'm almost done with the level," he called out. "Give me a second and I'll come over."

He heard Mama blow her nose and make noisy, deep in-and-out, jagged breaths. Jared knew level eighteen could wait. He got up and tossed the controller onto the sofa. He sat down at the kitchen table and immediately leaned back on his chair, waiting for the predictable motherly hand to settle him back down to all fours.

But it wasn't there.

He slowly lowered the chair himself. This was serious. His mother had gone back to dabbing her eyes with a shredded Kleenex. She reached over and tried to grab one of the napkins stuffed into the holder on the rotating tray in the middle of the table. Jared pulled out a napkin for her and several others with it. He quickly readjusted the pile with all corners stacked square and neat. He spoke up.

"Did something happen to Papa?"

"What? No. I mean, I don't know. That's not it."

Jared hadn't heard from his father in years but wasn't sure whether Mama still talked to him.

"I went to the doctor the other day."

"Mama? Are you sick or something?" Jared felt hot and his heart sped up.

"Well, some tests came back abnormal."

Mama often had a hard time getting to the point. Jared signaled with his hands for her to keep going. "It's OK, Mama. Just say it."

She took a deep breath in. "I might have cancer."

"What do you mean, you *might* have cancer?" Jared felt warm tears gathering in his eyes. He moved his hands under the table and started tapping his knees with his fingers, slowly at first, and then with more intention. It was another habit of his that Mama usually halted, often accompanied by a call to "stop the fidgeting." But this time, no comment.

Mama still hadn't responded.

"What kind of cancer?"

"Cervical cancer."

"Cervical? What's that?"

"The cervix . . . it's a girl part."

"What? Nooo." Jared waved his hand back and forth as if trying to erase the words from the air. "How do you get cancer of that?"

Mama sat up straight. "It comes from a virus. The reason I say that I might have cancer is because the doctor has to do more tests. I went to the gynecologist for a checkup and . . ."

"Mama, I can't . . . I can't hear about this right now." Jared didn't want Mama to see him cry. "I need to be alone for a little bit, OK?"

Mama nodded.

Safely inside his room, Jared crossed his arms and put his head down on his desk. He wanted to avoid crying. He tried to remember what he had learned in health class about the girl parts. Why didn't I pay more attention? he thought. He opened his laptop, got online, and searched for "cancer of the cervix."

Jared found information about the virus Mama had mentioned that could cause cervical cancer. It was called HPV, the human papillomavirus. He looked at drawings of a cervix. It looked like a bagel with a really small hole. He discovered the virus settled in the cells of the cervix and caused them to change. Sometimes the cells mutated so much that they became cancer. He thought about mutant aliens from his Xbox games and how freaky they looked. Jared wondered if the cervical cells looked freaky too and if that was how the doctors knew they weren't normal. There were hyperlinks to other articles. He read that a "Pap smear" was how women got tested for cervical cancer. That sounded uncomfortable: a doctor puts a thing in the vagina that looks like a duck beak so she can take a sample of cells from the cervix with a brush. Then there was "colposcopy," a biopsy of the cervix, and a "LEEP," a procedure that permanently removed pieces of the cervix.

Jared was overwhelmed. He had no idea women had to go through all this. The Internet said that cervical cancer could be prevented by a vaccine, along with regular pap smears. *So why did this happen, Mama*?

Jared came back out to the kitchen table with a sore neck and clenched jaw. Mama was sitting in the almost dusk of the kitchen. He turned on a light and sat down. He put his elbow on the table and rested his head in his hand. He traced invisible shapes with his other thumb over the wooden tabletop. Mama's eyes were puffy and red, but she had stopped crying.

"So, Mama." He swallowed. "I was reading about cervical cancer and Pap smears and stuff. Is that how they found out about you?"

"It is."

"So why didn't they find it sooner, on the other tests?"

Mama got up and went over to the sink. She turned to face Jared. "Well, my last Pap smear was when you were born."

"Mama! That was thirteen years ago. The Internet says you are supposed to get a Pap smear like every few years. Why didn't you?"

Mama came back over to Jared and, with that motherly force he knew well, put her hand on his shoulder. She went over to other side of the table, sat down, reached across, and held both of his hands in her own.

"Jared, it's not that simple. I didn't have health insurance for a long time. You do because you're young, but I didn't. I took a chance. We didn't have the money to spend on checkups for me. We needed money for rent and groceries and school supplies and clothes. It was stupid. I see that now. I should have found a way. But I didn't make it a priority. I never had a problem before. I thought I was being safe."

Jared looked away from Mama and over to the TV and wondered how many Xbox games it would take to pay for a Pap smear. Had he only known. He could have helped. All that birthday and holiday money spent on games. Mama's health was way more important that any stupid alien versus the universe challenge.

"Luckily, I have health insurance now with my job. So that's why I went for a checkup last week. I knew I was overdue. Jared, believe me, never in a million years would I have thought this would happen."

Mama pulled a piece of paper out of her purse and passed it to Jared. "This is what happens next. Tomorrow I go back to the doctor. I'm having this procedure, it's called a LEEP."

"Yeah, I read about that. They remove pieces of your cervix, right?" Then Jared thought about the duckbill thing and pieces of cervix and *maybe* cancer and he was scared. He knew Mama must be scared too. This was happening to her and to them.

"Does it hurt, the LEEP procedure?"

Mama shook her head confidently. "No. The doctor uses a numbing medicine so I won't feel anything. "

Jared nodded. He was glad because the duckbill thing sounded bad enough.

"Mama, does the duckbill thing hurt?"

Mama tilted her head and smiled. "You mean the speculum? No. If I was able to push you out, the weight and size of a small bowling ball, that's nothing."

Jared was relieved. For the first time that night he was hopeful. Maybe things really would be OK.

"Jared, before you go to bed, have everything ready for the morning. I'll have to drop you off early at school."

"I'll be up early, but I'm not going to school. I'm going with you tomorrow. You shouldn't have to go by yourself. This is too important."

"Jared, I wouldn't ask you to do that."

Jared smiled. "I know. You didn't." He hugged Mama. "Oh and by the way, I love you lots." Mama gladly hugged him back.

The next morning Jared got up two hours before he had to. Normally, he would have gone to school and normally if it weren't a school day he would have slept in, but since yesterday, nothing had happened normally. He wondered if things would ever be normal again.

Jared had never been to the gynecologist. Why would he? He walked into a room of women; a few men were there waiting with the women, but he was definitely the youngest person, girl or guy. He tried to imagine himself exploring a new world, or a new civilization, not the world of girl parts.

He sat down next to his mother. He looked through the magazines: *Working Mother, Cosmopolitan, Sports Illustrated, People*, and *Parents*. Not a single *Game Informer* among them. Jared chose *People* magazine, believing movie stars and celebrities to be the most interesting of them all. Besides, it seemed to be the magazine least likely to talk about the vagina, the cervix, the uterus, or the ovaries, all of the girl parts that had been reviewed in depth over the past twenty-four hours at home with Mama, on the Internet, and from the pamphlets the doctor had given her.

He did learn some important facts, though. The HPV vaccine hadn't been around for Mama, but he could get it. Viruses and cancer were way too microscopic for him. He wanted to point and shoot, search and destroy, not worry about things too small to see but so huge that they could change his life forever. With this vaccine, the virus couldn't touch him. No mutant cells for him.

Jared paged through two *People* magazines, one *Sports Illustrated*, and a *Cosmopolitan*. He thought that if he read the *Cosmopolitan*, he would get a deeper understanding about the world of girls, now that he knew their parts so well. He promised himself that if he ever found a girl he cared about, he would make sure she took care of her girl parts.

When he flipped through the magazines, he realized the girls in the magazines looked nothing like the girls he liked to spend time with. He liked girls who would play online *Star Force* or come over for hours of *Legend of Mutgut*. He liked girls who didn't mind playing video games with guys, not girls who cared about makeup and fashion and purses. He wanted their help to save the world by destroying one meechling at a time.

Soon, Mama joined him again in the waiting area. She said she felt fine and was glad it was over. It would be a week before she had the results.

It was about a week later when Mama came home later than usual. Jared was playing in the latest cyberspace challenge online. He heard the purse plop onto the counter. He heard the Macy's tag clink against the windowsill. He heard his mother settle into a kitchen chair. Then he heard faint crying.

She must have gotten her results, he thought.

Jared ran over to the table and sat down. "It's OK. Just say it. We'll figure out something."

"No. This is good. I'm good. No cancer. They removed everything and I should be fine. I'll follow up in six months and as often as I need to, until they say everything is negative. This is good news." Mama nodded her head and sighed. "All good."

Jared leaned over and put his arms around his mother's shoulders and hugged her until his back ached. "I love you, Mom."

Mama pulled back slightly and looked over to him. "Mom? I've never heard you call me that before.

"Yeah, well I never thought about you this way before. You're tougher than I realized. I mean, you're 'Mom,' able to overtake mutant, almost cancer, cells in a single shot. You're kinda awesome."

"Well, I've learned that everything else seems less important when you might or might not have cancer. You're a good son, Jared, and we're a good team."

"Thanks, Mom."

Mama tousled his hair. "I love you. Guy parts and all."

Jared couldn't speak. All the stress and worry and thought about a life without Mama was gone. It was his turn to cry.

So he did. And Mama hugged him back with tears in her eyes, with strength and protection that he had forgotten was there but gladly accepted.

Sabin Vaccine Institute
Kathy Wollner

The Sabin Vaccine Institute's mission is to reduce needless human suffering from vaccine-preventable and neglected tropical diseases. Sabin works toward its mission by developing new vaccines, advocating for increased use of existing vaccines, and promoting expanded access to affordable medical treatments.

Vaccines can prevent many illnesses, from the flu, as we learned in "A Pandemic Pig Tale," to HPV, as we learned in "Girl Parts." They work by giving your immune system, your body's defense against infection, a chance to recognize the virus or bacteria and therefore fight it off if you get exposed. Neglected tropical diseases are diseases that are uncommon in most parts of the world. They often affect the world's poor, and little money worldwide is spent on developing vaccines to prevent them or distributing medications to treat them. Vaccines are fundamental tools for warding off many of the diseases that exist in poor countries, such as polio. Scientists are continually working to develop better, more effective vaccines because preventing disease can be the most effective tool for improving community health in poor and rich countries alike.

Just like an illness can create hardship for a family, when disease is widespread in one place, it can challenge the development and progress of a whole country. Sabin believes that access to vital medicines and vaccines should be a basic service that governments guarantee for their people. Sabin works to spread awareness of neglected tropical diseases, their impact, and their prevention among populations and policy makers. It also seeks to develop and pass policies financing vaccine programs and developing funding mechanisms in various countries.

The Sabin Vaccine Institute Product Development Partnership (Sabin PDP) is the arm of the organization that focuses on creating safe, effective, low-cost vaccines for tropical infections in developing countries. It is more profitable for companies to develop vaccines for countries like the United States, where they can make money from the vaccine's development. But some of the greatest need for vaccines exists in the poorest regions of the world. Therefore, the Sabin PDP has collaborated with partners from across the globe to develop new, low-cost vaccines for diseases that primarily impact the world's poorest people, including human hookworm, schistosomiasis, and Chagas disease.

DISCUSSION QUESTIONS

- How are vaccines different from medicines?
- Can you think of some other diseases that are prevented by vaccines?
- How has scientific discovery improved disease-prevention efforts around the world?
- Name two barriers to getting medicines and vaccines that already exist to the people who need them.
- Where are most vaccines developed? Why is the Sabin PDP the only one working on vaccines for some of these diseases?
- What do you think would happen if, for example, schistosomiasis, a neglected tropical disease, was common in your community? How would the community and the government respond?

This section's information has been adapted from the Sabin Vaccine Institute's website. To learn more about Sabin and the vaccines they're working on, visit www.sabin.org.

Section VI

Health-Care Access

When people get sick, they need to access health care to diagnose and treat health problems. In many cases, people need access to a hospital to get the care they need. For example, if someone is in a car accident and has a ruptured internal organ, it is essential they get to a surgeon immediately. But not everyone lives close enough to a hospital, and in some countries, like the United States, where you have to pay for health care, not everyone can afford it. When thinking about health-care access, it is important to consider the three As: accessibility, availability, and affordability. In addition, without good, *quality* health care, accessibility, availability, and affordability cannot make a difference. Let's discuss these four important aspects of health-care access.

The first A is accessibility, which addresses how close someone lives to a health-care center and whether there are modes of transportation to help them get there. Living close to a health center may be someone's choice; perhaps they moved to live near a certain hospital because of a chronic illness or because they work in a hospital or community clinic. However, in most cases, the location of a health-care center is not a primary reason people move to a particular town or part of a city. Many people don't have the resources to move away from the community they were born into, and have limited choice in where they live. Nonetheless, where you live can shape your access to health services. For example, in small towns there's generally a primary health center but not always a hospital. Small hospitals located in towns usually serve many health problems but not all of them, and people with more complicated illnesses need to be sent to larger cities. Even within cities, there is varied access to hospitals. In some cases, people who live in wealthier areas of a city have access to more and better health centers and hospitals than people living in poorer areas of a city. Other problems exist, too, such as language barriers, which make it difficult for some patients (such as immigrants) to find health-care providers who can speak to them about their health problems.

The second A is availability. Even if a health center is nearby, it might not have the staff or equipment necessary to treat someone. This might be due to the fact that some health centers serve different purposes. A primary care community clinic would not generally be able to care for someone seriously injured in a car crash. This requires a higher level of care that is only available at larger hospitals. In the United States, hospitals that primarily take care of people who do not have insurance, such as safety-net hospitals, are often overwhelmed by the number of patients they serve. This means that people may wait a long time for a specialist appointment, a test to diagnose an illness, or a surgery because there are limited resources to serve many people.

The third A is affordability. Even if health care is accessible and available, it might not be affordable for some people. The affordability of health care differs between nations based on the type of health-care system. The United States has a market-based health-care system, and individuals have either private health insurance (usually through their employer) or government insurance if they qualify. Affordability of health care is a major issue that can be a barrier to people receiving the care they need. Because people have to pay for health care, people make choices about seeking care based on money rather than on whether they think they need help. In some cases, even if health care is accessible and available, people may not get care for their health problems because they cannot afford it. In "Girl Parts," Jared's mom's decided to delay care because she didn't have health insurance, illustrating how affordability can affect disease screening. This is not a system in which all people are treated equally. In contrast, the United Kingdom has a health-care system that is free for all citizens to access, meaning that it is not market based. Everyone has access to health-care services regardless of their ability to pay. These two systems are very different and shape the ways in which people seek and receive health care.

Finally, quality is a fundamental aspect of access to health care. You might have a health clinic that is accessible, where care is available and affordable, but without good, quality health care, it is possible that one might not get better. Quality is based on the training of the hospital staff, including clerks, nurses, doctors, and administrators, and the medications available to treat diseases. Quality also means that health-care providers are able to work with people from many different cultural and language backgrounds. Maintaining high-quality health care is an important part of ensuring that people place trust in the health-care system and believe that it is there to maintain health and treat illness in the best way possible.

This section describes the role of health-care access in people's health. We begin this section with "Scars," a story that highlights the tension of traditional beliefs, modern medicine, and mixed messages about public health interventions. "Mandy and the Motorized Wheelchair" demonstrates the important role of medical technology in improving the lives of people with disabilities. In "Open Secrets and Breaking Hearts," Mercedes becomes pregnant and must seek an unqualified person to carry out her abortion because in Peru it is against the law to terminate a pregnancy. Our final story, "There Will Always Be More Struggles to Win," shows how politics influence access to health care and how health workers can be critical to improving a community's health.

As you read through this section, consider the following questions:

- If you were injured, do you know where the closest medical center is located?

- Do you believe that you would receive high-quality care at the center you would visit? Why or why not?

- Would you go to a hospital or a clinic? Would there be staff available to care for you? Would this staff be trained well and be ready to take care of you? Would you be able to see a doctor or other health-care provider in a timely manner? Could you afford health-care treatments? Do you have private health insurance or a government health insurance?

- What influences quality of health care? Why is quality fundamental for the promotion of the three As?

23

Scars

Stephen Lavenberg

"Scars" is the story of Ronnie, a sixteen-year-old refugee in the United States who must confront his own cultural-identity issues in order to become an advocate for himself and his sick mzee *(grandfather). Since 1986, rebels called the Lord's Resistance Army have waged a war against the government of Uganda. Throughout this war, terrible atrocities have been committed against the people living in northern and eastern Uganda. In the late 1990s, when Ronnie and his mzee would have been leaving Uganda, the United Nations Office of the High Commissioner for Refugees documented well over two hundred thousand Ugandan refugees or internally displaced persons. This means they had lost their homes, and while some crossed into other countries, others were displaced inside of Uganda. Cultural and language barriers can lead to poor outcomes in health-care access and delivery. Health-care providers' understanding of cultural concepts or traditions relating to health can lead to more successful communication and therefore better outcomes. Tuberculosis (TB) is an illness caused by a bacteria that is both preventable and curable. It usually affects the lungs and is spread through the air by coughing. TB occurs in every*

part of the world, with most new infections found in Asia and sub-Saharan
Africa.

Ronnie woke up in the predawn darkness of his room. His mind was awake but his eyes were still closed, knowing it must be too early to get up. He heard a body-wracking cough from the next room. That must be what woke me up, he thought, his eyes still closed. He turned to look at the clock as the coughing continued from the other side of the thin wall. "Three thirty in the freaking morning," he muttered as he rolled out of bed. "Why?"

Ronnie shuffled to the doorway of the next room. The light from the streetlamp outside illuminated the outline of his grandfather sitting up at the edge of his bed.

"Mzee, are you all right? Do you need some water?" Ronnie asked. As his brain began to function, he remembered that even after twelve years in the United States, his grandfather, his mzee, still wasn't fluent in English. He quickly asked again in Ateso, the language of their village in Uganda.

"You sound terrible," Ronnie said with a weary voice as he handed his mzee a glass of water. "We should go to the clinic."

"No clinic!" his mzee shouted, breaking through the dark, half sleep where Ronnie was trying to remain. "It's just the flu. Get my medicine from Dr. Okino tomorrow and I'll be fine." He started a new fit of hacking coughs as he finished the last few words. Even in the dim light Ronnie could see his mzee's back muscles tense with each exertion; a shadow stood out on his left arm where Ronnie knew the skin was badly scarred from burns.

The shrieking beeps of his alarm clock jarred Ronnie back to consciousness three hours later. By 7:15 he was on his way to Westview Junior/Senior High School. On the way, he met up with Andrew and Patrick, his only friends. When his mzee brought him to America at the age of four, Ronnie was shy, but by the time he reached middle school, he had decided he was tired of being "the refugee" and made a conscious effort to "act American." Andrew and Patrick had dark skin like him, but they were born in the United States. They were what people referred to as African American, a term Ronnie never quite understood. Aren't I an African American? he thought. Regardless, Andrew and Patrick fit in and he didn't. He tried as hard as he could to be like them.

The class was told to quiet down as Mrs. Duncan stood next to a boy Ronnie had never seen before. "Good morning, everyone! I want you to give a warm welcome to the newest addition to our tenth-grade class," she said, smiling warmly at the tall black boy who stood next to her. "Welcome, Justin!"

"Whoa, do you see how dark he is?" whispered Patrick to Ronnie. "He's practically purple!" They both laughed as Mrs. Duncan went to her desk and Justin lumbered to his seat.

The rest of the day passed as usual: math, social studies, gym, lunch, science, then his double period in English. Ronnie hated English because he was in the remedial class, a double period intended to catch him up to the required tenth-grade reading level. Today they were discussing *The Old Man and the Sea*. He had a lot of trouble reading it.

"Ronnie," the teacher called, "what does Santiago think of the fish during his first day of fighting with it?"

"That fishing isn't worth his time?" he guessed.

"Hmm. Sam?"

"Santiago thinks of the fish like a brother, linked since they both have traveled really far out to sea," he said without hesitation. The other kids in class snickered and Ronnie caught someone whisper, "Dumb African can't learn" as he sank down into his seat.

I hate them, he thought. I wish I was born a genius so I could be in college now and not here with these stupid kids in this stupid school. I've lived in America almost my entire life and they still make fun of me for being from Africa. His eyes burned with anger.

"Psst! It's fine. Don't worry," said Justin.

"Shut up," snapped Ronnie, not wanting to be associated with the new kid, especially not another African.

After school, Ronnie, Andrew, and Patrick were playing basketball when Andrew asked about Justin. "Hey, I heard he is from Uganda too," he says. "Do you know him?"

"Yeah, can you speak jive with him?" Patrick joked.

Ronnie gritted his teeth. Andrew's question was innocent, but Patrick's sarcasm always seemed a bit more hostile than a friendly joke. Ronnie directed his answer to Andrew.

"His tribe is from northern Uganda, completely different from where my grandfather came from." He was careful to say "grandfather" instead of the respectful "mzee," and spoke of his grandfather's origin, not his own. He wanted to distance himself from the whole continent. Andrew seemed satisfied with the answer, but Patrick looked like he was gearing up for another teasing remark.

"I have to run, gotta pick up medicine for my grandfather," Ronnie interjected before Patrick could say anything.

Ronnie walked to the home of Dr. Okino, a small white house with faded-blue shutters and a matching faded-blue fence. Ronnie had known the doctor his entire life, so he was not surprised when he met him at the door wearing a leopard skin with his eyes bugging out beneath face paint and his hair matted up in dreadlocks. "*Biabo ijo, luapolon* [How are you, sir]? I'm just here for the medicine for my mzee," he announced through the screen.

"Ah, yes. He has bad spirits. The rainy season is a bad time for spirits. Make sure he puts this powder into his tea every evening," Dr. Okino whispered as he handed Ronnie a jar filled with a dark-green powder.

Ronnie rolled his eyes as he walked away. Dr. Okino was a witch doctor. He did not try to hide it, and everyone in the community knew. He looked crazy when he answered the door, but he was the only doctor Ronnie's mzee would see.

When Ronnie entered the house, his mzee was asleep in his favorite tattered green faux-suede chair, the radio still playing the BBC. Who even listens to the radio anymore? he asked himself for the millionth time. His mzee, that was who. Twelve years ago he had brought Ronnie and his radio to the United States. They left behind Ronnie's parents, three brothers, and two sisters, and the rest of their belongings. Some days, after school, Ronnie would sit with his mzee and listen to the radio—BBC news from around the world.

Then one day they heard a report come in about a camp in Uganda. They called them internally displaced persons, or IDP, camps, for people who had to leave their homes because they were unsafe or had been destroyed. Ronnie was only six at the time, but he knew something had happened. Tense whispers circled through the community at church. The government, tasked with protecting the camp, had actually attacked it. Maybe it was rebels dressed as government soldiers—nobody could be sure. Women and children were raped, the feet of every man and boy were lopped off with machetes, and everything was burned. Ronnie wasn't allowed to listen to the radio after that, and his mzee stopped talking about their family. The members of the church, who were all Ugandan except for one Tanzanian family, became their family. They were the people Ronnie and his mzee invited over for tea, the people whose houses Ronnie and his mzee went to for Christian or Ugandan celebrations. All the men and women became "uncles" and "aunties" and their children Ronnie's cousins.

His memory faded as he came back to the present. He stood in the kitchen as the milk boiled on the stove. He turned the gas off, added the tea leaves and sugar, and placed the dark-green powder bag next to his mzee's cup before he woke him up.

The next few weeks in school Ronnie tried to lay low. He focused on his English homework and spent a lot of time with Patrick and Andrew. A few times Justin tried to talk to him or sit with him at lunch, but Ronnie avoided him. He didn't want to associate with Justin and certainly didn't want to give Patrick any reason to make fun of him. Sometimes Ronnie thought Justin understood, but he still kept away from situations where Justin might have taken the chance to talk to him. Ronnie didn't want anything to do with him.

By springtime Ronnie was exhausted from waking up early each morning to his mzee's hacking cough. The dark-green powder didn't seem to be working, and the cough had gone on too long to be the flu.

"Mzee, go to the clinic and get a checkup. It has been three months and you don't seem any better," Ronnie said softly to him as he got ready to leave for school.

"No," he replied with barely concealed anger. "Those Western doctors hate our people. They hate our black skin. They are trying to kill us. When you go in they insist on giving you an injection. Giving everyone an injection. Well, you know what? Those injections make you unable to make a baby! That's what they do! I've seen it with my own eyes! They kill us off by making us think we are getting medicine but instead they destroy us by preventing our people from reproducing. They even"—his tone quieted down to a conspiratorial whisper—"made AIDS to kill all the Africans." He grabbed Ronnie's arm tight and pulled him close as he started to turn out the door. "You be careful, Ronnie. The white man made AIDS to kill us Africans, and they are ruthless. Don't let anyone trick you!"

"OK," Ronnie mumbled as he pulled away. *Geez, what a way to start the day.*

Later, as he sat in English class, the teacher asked for a volunteer to read. Nobody raised a hand. This was how it went every day, and every day the teacher ended up picking someone. Since he had been doing better in class, Ronnie knew the teacher would not call on him. "Justin," the teacher said, "the top of page 42." Justin stuttered and tried to read the words before the teacher asked him to stop.

"Justin?" the teacher asked.

"Yes?"

"Do you want to try again?"

Justin fell into complete silence. The students around him started to snicker. Whispers started about the "stupid African." Justin looked at Ronnie with imploring eyes. Ronnie couldn't stand it and he looked away.

After class, Andrew, Patrick, and Ronnie were at their lockers. They were finished for the day and Ronnie just wanted to get out of there. He was haunted by the look in Justin's eyes and ashamed at how he said nothing. The hairs on the back of his neck perked up when he heard Patrick whisper Justin's name. What was Ronnie supposed to do? Andrew and Patrick were supposed to be his friends. He forced a laugh as Patrick cracked a joke about Justin's gangly frame and awkward walk.

A few pickup games of basketball after school helped calm Ronnie's nerves. On his way home he had to run to Dr. Okino's house. He had almost forgotten to pick up the medicine for his mzee. This time, Dr. Okino was dressed a bit less eccentrically, so Ronnie felt less hesitant. He decided to ask Dr. Okino a few questions about the dark-green powder he gave to treat Ronnie's mzee.

"What is this stuff?"

"It is made from the Artemisia plant and is mixed with *tungawusi*," he said, using the Ateso word for ginger.

"But my mzee isn't getting any better."

"He has not sacrificed to the spirits."

"Right." This was going nowhere, so Ronnie thanked him and left.

He walked into his house and stopped. Justin was sitting at the kitchen table with a hot cup of tea, across from Ronnie's mzee, who beckoned him to bring the medicine. He sat and sipped his tea in silence as Justin and his mzee talked. Ronnie realized his mzee understood some of the language from the north.

In Uganda, tea is more than just a beverage. It is a humble offering to a guest, a reason to spend forty minutes talking with friends or neighbors. And usually, it happens when you least expect it. While his mzee and Justin talked, Ronnie sat in silence, fulfilling his role as a respectful host by being present, although he silently wished every moment that Justin would just get out of his house. Finally the time came. As Ronnie walked him to the door, Justin turned and said, "I think your mzee is very sick."

"I know that. Who do you think has been getting him his medicine?" Ronnie said, irritated and aching for him to leave.

"He coughed some blood into his handkerchief," Justin said softly.

"Yeah, I know," Ronnie quickly responded, not wanting to let the fear of this news enter his voice. He needed to change the subject. "How come you can't read?"

Justin hung his head in shame. "I can read, kind of. The teacher says I have 'functional illiteracy.' I can speak but I can't read anything complex or write much. I never learned." He looked up. "You need to get your mzee to the clinic, Ronnie."

He turned and walked away. Ronnie watched as Justin became illuminated under the streetlights and faded almost to nothing in the darkness between them.

Ronnie woke up in the predawn darkness of his room. His mind was awake but his eyes were still closed, knowing it must be too early to get up. He heard the body-wracking cough from the next room. It sounded worse.

"Mzee, we need to get you to the clinic," he said.

"No, take me to Dr. Okino."

In the wee hours of the morning, Ronnie half-walked, half-carried his mzee to the small white house with faded-blue shutters and a matching faded-blue fence. Dr. Okino welcomed them inside and led them to a bedroom he had converted into what appeared to be a ceremonial room. Ronnie had heard about them from his mzee, but had never seen one in person. He thought they were a thing of the past. One of Dr. Okino's weary-eyed sons sat on the floor, his legs wrapped around a wooden drum with a goatskin cover.

What followed next sent Ronnie's head spiraling. The boy started drumming. Dr. Okino lit candles and strange-smelling herbs that gave off a smoke that burned Ronnie's eyes. Dr. Okino sat down with Ronnie's mzee in front of a large wooden bowl. Together they started chanting to the beat hammered out by the boy.

We go to church every Sunday, Ronnie thought. What is this? The pulsating beat pushed the thoughts out of his head. His senses were overcome with the pounding of the drum, his nose filled with the scent of the herbs, and his eyes watered from the smoke. Through the tears and haze he thought he saw a dark, thick liquid filling the wooden bowl.

He squinted and tried to wave the smoke out of his face, but his view was blocked by how his mzee was sitting. Is this the sacrifice to the spirits? he thought. His mzee drank from the bowl, and the whirlwind of activity was over as quickly as it had begun. Dr. Okino helped Ronnie raise his mzee to standing, and soon he was once again half-walking, half-carrying the old man through the cool morning air.

School that day was a daze. Ronnie floated from one class to the next overwhelmed and disturbed by what had happened that morning. Absentmindedly chewing on his lunch, he was brought crashing down to earth as he saw Justin walking toward him.

"Hey Ronnie, how's your mzee?"

"Well, well! Ronnie, your African brother is here to talk to you," Patrick chuckled. He put on a serious face and continued, "Click click, ahh click dok ching chong." He managed to keep his face straight for two seconds before he burst out laughing, his whole body collapsing in on itself.

The rage exploded inside of Ronnie. Andrew pulled Patrick back and Justin grabbed Ronnie just before he landed on Patrick, throwing punches within inches of his face. "What? You think your black skin is better than mine?" Ronnie shouted into Patrick's face, each word dripping with anger. "You think the fact that your ancestors were slaves makes you better than me, coming straight from Africa because my people were being slaughtered? You think people don't notice that your grades aren't any better than mine? For years I put up with your crap because I thought if I acted American enough, if I acted like you we could be friends and I could be accepted. Now I realize you only see differences and the next opportunity to put someone down."

Patrick shook loose from Andrew's hold, his eyes wide as he looked from Ronnie to Justin then back to Ronnie again. He turned and stormed off. Andrew looked at Ronnie and whispered, "I'm sorry" before he ran after Patrick.

Ronnie was exhausted. He felt like he had just lost his only friends, and his mind was still a jumble from the voodoo-like happenings at Dr. Okino's. Before Justin could say anything, Ronnie walked away.

The rest of the day passed in a fog. Luckily it was easy for Ronnie to avoid everyone. On his way home, he couldn't stop replaying all the events of the day in his head. The feeling of finally having stood up to Patrick made him realize he needed to continue to take action. He would go to the clinic and schedule an appointment, he decided. Then he'd worry about getting his mzee there.

The community clinic was simultaneously sterile and full of life. The walls, floors, chairs—every surface—was a dull pink or blue, almost gray. The waiting room was half-full with people of all different colors and sizes. They waited in chairs while young children entertained themselves nearby. The sight made the place come alive. Some people were dressed in colorful prints from their native countries while others brought lively chatter in a variety of languages. As Ronnie walked to the front to make an appointment, he caught sight of a woman he recognized from church. She was wearing scrubs and sat behind a desk with a headset on.

"Hello, Miss Belinda."

"Ronnie! Nice to see you. You don't look sick—are you here to schedule an appointment?"

"Sort of," he replied. "It's an appointment for my mzee. He has been coughing for months now, but he won't come to the clinic." He told her about the powder and that he had coughed up blood. "I'm worried about him."

"Ah, I see," Belinda said. She seemed to understand his conundrum. "I have an idea."

At dinner that night, Ronnie told his mzee he had run into a woman from church who invited them over for tea the next day. Ronnie knew his mzee would not be able to refuse an invitation for tea.

🔳

The next evening they knocked on the door of a quaint little apartment. A tall Kenyan man opened the door, invited them in, and introduced himself as Isaac, Belinda's husband. Ronnie's mzee and Isaac exchanged the traditional greetings, a ritual that always seemed longer than necessary, even when you knew the person. After introductions, they all headed into the small kitchen, where Ronnie could smell ginger and spices coming from the boiling milk.

Isaac left them to tend to one of his children while Ronnie and his mzee remained in the kitchen with Belinda. Ronnie felt awkward because no one was speaking. Sitting in Belinda's kitchen, his mzee looked old. His back was hunched over and his eyes were weary. It was time to put their plan into action.

"Belinda, where do you work?" he asked, trying to sound casual.

"At the community clinic," she said. "I trained as a nurse at Mulago Hospital in Uganda, but I'm not qualified to work as a nurse in the United States, so I just do scheduling and basic office work."

"Wow, that's interesting." Too much? Ronnie thought. He went on to describe his mzee's cough to Belinda, as he had the day before. Just as expected, his mzee chimed in at the intended moment. He told Belinda that Dr. Okino gave him some herbal medicine and he felt much better. Belinda explained that the herbal medicine Dr. Okino gave Ronnie's mzee was good, that it actually was what was used to treat malaria.

"But there is no malaria in the United States," she continued. "And I think you should be tested for tuberculosis." She pulled some pamphlets from the shelf and brought them to the table.

"Thank you very much. We should really be going now," his mzee said.

Tea was an ordeal, yet there they were, fifteen minutes in, and his grandfather wanted to leave. His mzee looked at Ronnie as he stood, and in his eyes Ronnie caught a glimpse of the same look Justin had when the teacher had asked him to read in class. They took the pamphlets as Belinda's husband came back to wish them farewell.

It was a quiet walk home. When they got inside, his mzee put the pamphlets on top of the pile of junk mail. Ronnie understood now why they had left Belinda's. His mzee was ashamed. It dawned on Ronnie that he had never seen his mzee read. Ronnie knew his mzee never learned much English, but he had never even seen him with the Ateso newspapers that circled around the neighborhood. He didn't use a Bible at church and never went on the computer. He didn't travel far, but when he did, he never used a map but just asked for directions. He always listened to the radio. Suddenly it all made sense.

"Mzee, why don't we read these pamphlets together?" Since they got them from a nurse trained in a Ugandan hospital, he thought his mzee might be willing to take a chance.

"OK," his mzee said as he sat down. Ronnie's heart surged with joy.

An hour later they had read each pamphlet, and it seemed to Ronnie that his mzee fit every description of someone who suffered from tuberculosis.

"Great, so let's make an appointment at the clinic for a test," Ronnie proposed.

"No," his mzee said, his fingers absentmindedly touching the scars on his upper arm.

Ronnie was so confused and frustrated.

His mzee continued, "Let me tell you, Ronnie. In Uganda we suffered. It was a struggle to live under the regime and we almost died escaping to Kenya. Two rebels caught us. They put a machete in the fire then started slapping it against my arm. I passed out from the wretched pain. If it had not been for the bravery of the other men we traveled with, we wouldn't be here today. Once we got to the refugee camp in Kenya, things seemed to improve. There was food, shelter. It was meager, but at least you and I were together, at least we were alive. The white foreigners came and brought us rice and beans and oil to cook with. They brought us blankets and even set up a school for the youth. Then they started bringing in the young doctors. The doctors saved my burned arm from infection—that was good. But then, each person had to go in to see the doctor and each person got at least one injection, most got many. They didn't tell us what they were."

Ronnie listened with awe.

"A few weeks after that people started dying," his mzee continued. "They said it was from poor diet. They said we were sick before we got there. They said they had more medicine for us. But the truth was that they were killing us. I won't go to these young Western doctors."

His mzee got up and went to sleep while Ronnie mulled over all this new information.

Over the next few weeks Ronnie started talking to Justin more. They started hanging out during lunch and even after school. Justin was Ronnie's first true friend. They supported each other and looked out for each other. It made Ronnie ashamed to think he had been so mean to Justin, but he made up for it each chance he got. Ronnie was proud to have Justin as a friend.

One day at lunch Ronnie brought up the story his mzee had told him about the scar. "How do I get my mzee to the clinic?"

Justin smiled with sad eyes. "These things happen in the camps, the death and disease. It happened in the one I was in. The reality is not quite what your mzee thought. The doctors were giving vaccines to prevent disease. It is true that some young children were so malnourished they died because they couldn't absorb the nutrients in the food. During the conflict, many women were raped by the rebels or by the soldiers. The women would get infections, even HIV, but they didn't tell their husbands out of fear or shame. The infections spread and eventually babies were born with malformations. People blamed the doctors because they didn't understand the illnesses. The truth is that it was our own people who were killing us."

"So what can I possibly do? There must be a way I can get my mzee help," Ronnie said.

"Why not go and get an appointment with an older doctor? You speak English so they can communicate with you. You could make sure your appointment is with an older male doctor."

"But what if he's right?" Ronnie said. "I know so many families who refuse to go to the clinic because they say the doctors assume all refugees have AIDS. What if I bring him there and they treat him badly?"

"Those families are just covering up for their inability to understand the information the doctors give them. They are functional illiterates like me. You can't see it, but I know the tricks for covering it up, so I can tell."

After school, Ronnie walked to the clinic and waited for Belinda. Together they scheduled an appointment with an older doctor.

At dinner Ronnie told his mzee, "We are going to the clinic this week." Before he could interrupt, Ronnie went on, "I made you an appointment with an older doctor. Mzee, I'm afraid of losing you. We learned a few weeks ago that tuberculosis can be treated, but you could die if it's not. For all these years you have worked hard and taken care of me. What would happen if I lost you now?" Ronnie saw the effect of his words as his mzee started to consider the idea.

"OK," was all he said.

A few days later, they were at the clinic. Ronnie's mzee was very nervous and tense. He saw Belinda and took the usual five minutes to go through all the traditional greetings with her. Ronnie could tell his mzee was relaxing as each pleasantry was exchanged. She assured him of the skill and experience of the doctor, and he took her words easily.

In the exam room, Ronnie's mzee was quiet while the doctor asked questions and Ronnie answered. Mostly Ronnie interpreted the doctor's words and his mzee nodded in acceptance. Much of what the doctor said, though, Ronnie had trouble understanding. Chest x-ray? Sputum? Microscopy testing? Progression of illness? Contagious? Ronnie asked many questions until the doctor had explained each point in simple words that Ronnie felt confident he could comprehend and interpret. The doctor gave them a mask and told him his mzee should wear it anytime he was outside the house. As they walked out of the clinic, Ronnie felt exhausted. The experience was stressful, but he felt that the effort was worthwhile. He felt there was hope for his mzee.

At school the next day, Ronnie was excited to relay every bit of the experience to Justin. They talked about it during lunch and Ronnie told him how thankful he was for his help.

"You did all the work," he reminded Ronnie. "I'm happy to hear that your mzee is going to get help."

That night, as his mzee and he were about to start cooking, the phone rang. It was a woman who introduced herself as a nurse who works with the doctor they had seen.

"Your grandfather's test results came back, and he does have tuberculosis," she said. "The doctor would like you to come in with your grandfather to go over his treatment. Can I make him an appointment for tomorrow?"

Ronnie relayed this to his mzee. He nodded grimly. Ronnie explained to the nurse that the appointment would need to be in the afternoon after school was out. Thankfully, she was able to squeeze them in just before closing.

Ronnie called Justin and told him that the test was positive.

"Why don't you and your mzee come over for dinner tonight?" Justin asked.

Ronnie was more than happy to accept. At Justin's house, they shared the meal with his family and only briefly talked about the call. Everyone agreed that the appointment the next day would tell them what they needed to know, and until then, there was nothing they could do but enjoy the delicious food Justin's mom had prepared. Ronnie felt the relief grow with each bite of food. He was so thankful he didn't have to go through this alone.

The next day at the clinic, the doctor rushed through their visit. He explained everything quickly and didn't give Ronnie time to ask questions before he moved on to his next patient. There were so many medicines with different instructions. He was overwhelmed and frustrated he didn't get the information he needed to explain everything to his mzee. On their way out, Belinda caught them. "You look shell shocked," she said. "Why don't you come back to my house and have dinner?"

Over another tasty dinner of traditional millet bread and sesame-pasted fish stew they talked through the confusion. Belinda was kind and patient and explained each component of the treatment process and answered their questions. Ronnie could tell his mzee was worried about the intensity of the treatment.

"Why are there so many medicines for just one illness?" he asked. But having everything explained directly in a language he understood helped him relax. He trusted Belinda, so he was all right with the doctor's plan.

▦

Ronnie woke up in the predawn darkness of his room. His mind was awake but his eyes were still closed, knowing it must be too early to get up. He turned to look at the clock. "Three thirty in the freaking morning," he muttered under his breath. "Why am I awake?" He strained his ears and heard nothing but the sound of his own breathing. Ronnie smiled, turned over, and went back to sleep.

The shrieking beeps of his alarm clock jarred him back to consciousness three hours later. By 7:15 a.m., he and his mzee were headed to church. Afterward, they went with Justin and his family and Belinda and her family to the park to celebrate Martyr's Day.

Ronnie's mzee, cleared of tuberculosis, played with Belinda's young children. The joy in his eyes didn't diminish one bit when the young toddler he was holding started to poke the scars on his upper arm. Ronnie looked at the scene and was filled with great joy and thanks. Through the strength of their bonds, they had enabled each other to reach that amazing day. Justin finished the year almost caught up in English, though he would have to take a double period again the next year, but tutoring Justin had helped Ronnie so much that he would only have to take one. I am proud to be part of this family, Ronnie thought. Together we are embracing the scars life has given us.

24
Mandy and the Motorized Wheelchair

Patrick Klacza

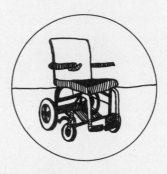

"Mandy and the Motorized Wheelchair" tells the story of a young woman with cerebral palsy (CP), a motor condition that affects a person's ability to move. Cerebral palsy is almost always congenital, meaning it comes about or at the time of birth, so people with CP have lived with their physical disabilities their whole lives. This story illustrates the difficulties of living with a disability in the United States and demonstrates the impact of medical technology on independence and productivity for people with disabilities. We follow Mandy as she gets a new wheelchair that allows her to better get around and pursue her independence. Despite her rigid limbs, Mandy secures a job at the local library and finds a new source of self-confidence.

Simon was late again. There were too many broken wheelchairs in Illinois for one man to fix, getting him on the phone was impossible, and maybe he wouldn't come. Mandy had to leave voicemails, and she wasn't good on the phone. She articulated poorly, and her messages went unanswered.

But Mandy couldn't wait another day. Her new chair was parked in the corner of the bedroom, and she had barely practiced driving it. She'd scored a job interview at the public library, and she needed to be able to get around. She couldn't shelve books with someone pushing her, now could she?

Mandy's aunt had rushed to buy the new wheelchair. The money from the government was there, and if she'd waited, it could've been snatched away. She went into the store and told the salesman about Mandy and how she needed a motorized wheelchair to get around. The salesman pointed her toward the second-most expensive chair on the floor, one with many buttons and triggers and a computer screen. Her aunt, feeling overwhelmed and pressured by the clerk, said, "I'll take it" and wheeled it out that very day.

Now it sat in the corner.

The buttons were all wrong. Forward/reverse should've been up by Mandy's temple so she could toggle it on and off with her head. The driver's joystick was supposed to be near her armpit, where she could reach it. It was tough living with cerebral palsy. Her classmate Jason also had it, and he walked with a bad limp. He called it a swagger, though, and yeah it sucked, but he still got to walk. She'd never walk. Not fair.

Finally, an hour later, Simon the wheelchair guy came. He started fixing Mandy's chair. He moved buttons with a screwdriver and asked Mandy how they felt.

"They feel fine," she said.

"And how about this?" he asked, fixing the joystick.

"That feels fine too."

"You know you can make these changes yourself."

"How can I make them?"

"Oh, not you," he said. "Your aunt can make them. All she needs is a screwdriver."

"Oh."

He didn't stay more than ten minutes. Mandy's aunt did try to fix the chair herself, but Simon had screwed those screws in so darn tight so she'd have to call him and pay him because he was the only one who could unscrew them, that crook.

Mandy powered up and shifted into gear. She fingered the joystick and inched ahead. At first she moved slowly and with jerks, but she eventually drove smoothly around her kitchen table and into her bedroom. It was her first real taste of freedom since the last time Simon was there. She hoped it would last.

For the job interview, Mandy chose a smart ensemble. She couldn't wear heels, though. Her feet wouldn't fit into them. She wanted to go alone, but her aunt had to come along to push, listen to the details, and interpret. Strangers didn't always understand Mandy's speech. Her cerebral palsy affected the muscles in her mouth just like the ones in her legs.

The interviewer, an older lady in pink, asked easy questions at first. "How come you want to work at the library?"

Mandy said, "I love books and want steady work."

"What?"

"I love books and want steady work," she repeated.

"What?"

"I love books!"

The interviewer's glasses about fell off. "That's good," she said. "I love books too." She read Mandy's resume one last time. "I'll hire you, but only under one condition. You must come to work alone. You'll need to use your electric wheelchair."

Mandy wanted to jump, but couldn't of course, and instead moved her tense arms as much as possible, sort of like her version of the fist pump. This resulted in painful muscle spasms. She knew she had a long way to go if she ever wanted to be a good librarian.

The day before Mandy was supposed to start, her chair broke. She was stuck on the slowest speed. It took a full minute to get from one end of the apartment to the other. How long would it take in the vast library? Naturally, she panicked.

"What if we can't fix it?" she asked her aunt.

"We'll fix it, sweetie."

"What if my boss fires me?"

"So then she fires you. You can find a new job."

"But I don't want a new job."

Before it was time to go, Mandy's aunt kissed Mandy on the cheek. She straightened her clothes. Her back was killing her—it was always killing her—but she bent over to fix Mandy's footrest. The chair was still broken.

"Can't you do anything?" Mandy asked.

"I've tried. I screwed the loose screws, charged the battery, whacked the buttons. What more do you want from me?"

"Check near the wheels."

"Wait a minute. You might be onto something!" Just then, Mandy's aunt saw the problem: a hidden, frayed wire. She rushed into the kitchen and returned with the roll of duct tape. She wrapped the frayed part of the wire. "Try it now."

Mandy moved the joystick. The chair jolted forward and scared the bejeezus out of her aunt. Mandy sped around the kitchen table, testing her chair for glitches. "How did you do that?" she asked.

"I think I just proved once and for all that duct tape fixes everything."

A crowd of library employees watched Mandy from the main desk. She had a small stack of books on her lap and was about to make her first attempt at shelving. Her chair moved effortlessly. The practice, for now, had paid off.

"C'mon, Mandy," said Maude, one of the librarians.

"Oh, she can do it," said another named Helen.

"Look at that wheelchair. It's like a spaceship."

"It's like a car."

Mandy turned into an aisle and scanned the shelves. Her first book's barcode said FAU. It was William Faulkner's *The Sound and the Fury*. Mandy looked up. Faulkner's place was high on the shelf. She'd need to reach for this one.

"C'mon, Mandy," said Maude.

"C'mon, Mandy," said Helen.

Mandy put her left arm up. The book was in her hand, the shelf still inches away. She dug her heels in and pushed. Her butt came off the seat. She was nearly there.

"Should I help her?"

"Just wait. She can do it."

"I hate to see her strain like that."

"She strains because she wants to do the job right."

Mandy was so close. She moved her spastic arm so that it was almost straight and pushed with all her might. Not even her physical therapist could get her to do that. The book's spine was on the shelf now, but the rest of the book still hung perilously. The other librarians weren't working at all anymore but watching Mandy's every move. A boy said hello, and they shushed him in unison. Mandy was shaking now, but she would not spasm. She would not give in. It was only one book, but it was her first book, and she was going to get it on that shelf. Because that was her job, and she would perform it to the best of her ability. Her boss wouldn't regret hiring her. She had a motorized wheelchair that worked, she had a book, and she had her body. All she needed was one more push.

The book slid onto the shelf in perfect alphabetical order. Mandy sank back into her wheelchair with a whoosh and smiled. A bead of sweat fell from her hair. She had done it. The librarians let out a cheer. They came over to congratulate her—to pat her on the back—but she waved them away.

"Thanks, but I've still got a job to do." Mandy picked up the second book in her stack—William Golding's *Lord of the Flies*—and drove over to the Gs. The way she saw it, she had only just begun to work.

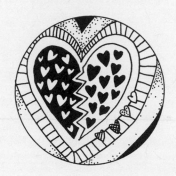

25
Open Secrets and Breaking Hearts

Heather Wurtz

"Open Secrets and Breaking Hearts" introduces the challenges women face when they are unable to access safe abortion care. Abortion, or pregnancy termination, is a procedure that can be performed very safely by a trained health professional in a clinic or hospital. However, according to the World Health Organization, a woman dies from complications of unsafe abortions every eight minutes. Ninety-seven percent of these cases take place in developing countries with highly restrictive abortion laws. This story follows Mercedes's experience seeking an abortion from a provider who is not a trained health-care professional. Unsafe abortions can lead to many problems due to blood loss, infection, and physical trauma, and they can even result in death. It is often the most vulnerable women, like Mercedes—young, poor, and marginalized—who suffer the greatest consequences. This story teaches us the impact of policies on health-care access and health outcomes and how women's openness and honesty about their own experiences can educate and inspire others.

Katia held Mercedes's hand tightly and soothingly brushed her hair away from her forehead. Mercedes's voice shook. "I can't have a baby," she said, crying. "It's impossible. No tengo opción [I don't have a choice]."

Katia pulled Mercedes into a hug. Mercedes had been her best friend since they had arrived in Lima, Peru, nearly three years ago. Like Katia, Mercedes came to Lima from a small rural pueblo (town) to work as a live-in nanny and housekeeper for a wealthy family. Mercedes moved into a neighboring building only a few weeks after Katia moved in with her señora. They frequently saw each other at the nearby park where they took the children to play. Katia remembered the first afternoon at the park when they first started to get to know each other.

"So what do you think of Lima?" Katia had said, after shooing the children away to go play with the others.

"It's OK, I suppose," replied Mercedes, with a moment of hesitation. "But I really miss my mama. She must be so busy now with no one to help with my little brother and sisters."

"Why did you move here when you are so needed at home?" asked Katia.

"Well," said Mercedes, "I am able to make much more money working here in Lima than what our small farm at home can bring in, especially since my papa died last year. There have been so many nights since then when we've barely had enough to eat. Mama would sometimes skip dinner so my little siblings could have larger servings. She said they were young and growing and needed it more than she did." Mercedes gave Katia a small smile, although Katia could see sadness in her eyes.

"When my aunt phoned Mama and told her that she knew a family looking for a girl to keep house in the city," Mercedes went on, "I couldn't turn the position down. My wages are enough to feed my family every night. By being in the city, I hope I might have the chance to get an education. If I save enough money each month, I could start night school if it's OK with the señora. I've always wanted to be a teacher."

Katia nodded her head in agreement. "Yes, education is the best way to *superar* [get ahead in life]. Especially if you can learn to fit in with the urbanites, with their refined Spanish and modern clothes." She imitated the wealthy women who lived in the neighborhood where they worked. Mercedes laughed.

"Yes," said Mercedes, her eyes brightening with hope. "Do you really think I could be like them?"

Since that afternoon, Katia and Mercedes often spent their days off together. Mercedes had almost saved enough money to begin school. Now all that she had worked for was on the brink of being lost.

"If the señora finds out that I am pregnant, she will fire me on the spot!" Mercedes said, wiping away her tears with her sleeve. "How can I work as a nanny with a child of my own to care for? And I don't even know what's become of Fernando! The last time I saw him he said he was going to leave Peru to find work in Costa Rica. He won't be here to help me raise a child. And what will my family do? They are all relying on me!"

Katia hesitated, feeling her own sense of internal conflict.

"Look, my cousin knows someone who can take care of it, if that's what you want. I will find out where to go. But you'll need to bring some money."

Mercedes started to cry again. "I never thought I'd be in this position." She nodded her head and quickly dried her eyes. "I can bring the money."

On Sunday, their day off, Mercedes and Katia met at the park. Mercedes's long black hair was pulled back into a braid, and she wore jeans with a purple blouse beneath a black cardigan. She looked surprisingly calm.

"Maybe if I look put together," she said, "I'll trick myself into feeling it."

Katia and Mercedes caught a *cumbi* (shared van) to their destination, and Katia led Mercedes down a long alleyway to the address she'd marked on a small notepad in her pocket. After a quick knock on the door, an older woman answered and led them to the back of the apartment. The woman asked them to sit down and wait for the señor and then disappeared, leaving them alone. Katia looked over at Mercedes and noticed small drops of sweat on her brow. Her hands were shaking and her face was pale. The silence was nearly unbearable.

"I'm scared, Katia," she whispered.

A man appeared and Mercedes handed him the payment, nearly half her monthly salary. He told Mercedes to follow him but stopped Katia when she rose to come along.

"Just her," he said abruptly. Fear in her eyes, Mercedes gave Katia one last long look before she disappeared with the señor behind the closed door.

Katia waited and waited, her anxiety building. "This is taking too long," she said to herself. She began pacing and fidgeting with her hands. Something did not feel right. Finally the man emerged, looking exasperated and unsteadied.

"You must get her out of here," he said. "She is still bleeding, but there is no more that I can do."

"Qué dice? [What are you saying?]" Katia shouted. He pushed her toward the room. "Take her!" he shouted again, becoming more agitated.

Katia opened the door and stepped into the stuffy, poorly lit room. A pungent odor of bodily liquids overwhelmed her and she nearly vomited. She saw Mercedes lying on a narrow metal table. She was very still and very pale. Beneath the table, Katia realized with horror, a pool of blood was collecting on the concrete floor. A sink in the corner of the room was littered with metal tools and bloody latex gloves. A wastebin overflowed with blood-soaked tissues and saturated pads of gauze.

"You must go!" the man shouted again. He was scared, Katia realized, scared of what he had done and could not fix.

She heard Mercedes groan—a deep, visceral cry of anguish. Katia went to her side and, with difficulty, helped her off the table. She partly walked her and partly dragged her out of the apartment. Katia's heart pounded in her chest and she began to cry as Mercedes became heavier in her arms and started to drift in and out of consciousness. They finally made it onto the street.

"Ayudanos! [Help us!]" Katia cried out, searching for a sympathetic stranger. Katia's legs buckled beneath her, her energy waned, and they both sunk to the ground.

She heard somebody call for an ambulance and felt a hand lock beneath her arm to try to keep her upright. Although a whirlwind of movement had set in all around her, she felt like the world had suddenly come to a disastrous halt. She closed her eyes for a minute of relief.

◼

Katia was by Mercedes's side when she woke in the hospital. She had brought soup for Mercedes for when she could eat. After her surgery, Mercedes began receiving fluids through an intravenous (IV) tube in her arm. Katia looked around the room. There were several beds with patients, each separated by a tattered green curtain. The thinly padded, metal-framed hospital bed reminded Katia of the man's abortion table, and her heart jumped at the horrifying memory. The bright lights and the constant beeping, buzzing, and other commotion around her made her feel like she was in another world.

"Gracias a Dios [thanks to God] you are here, Katia," Mercedes said. "I feel like I've been hit by a truck. And I'm so thirsty." She licked her chapped lips. "My belly hurts so badly, and every time I breathe it gets worse. What happened to me?"

A doctor approached, wearing a long white coat, a stethoscope around her neck, and a somber expression on her face. "I'm not going to ask any questions," stated the doctor, in a neutral tone. "But you should know that you almost died. You lost so much blood we had to give you a transfusion." She paused. "And we had to remove your uterus, Mercedes, to save your life. I'm afraid that you won't be able to have children.

Whoever was trying to help you put a hole in your uterus. You got anti-biotics in your IV to keep you from developing an infection. We're going to keep you here to make sure you improve. Do you have any questions right now?"

Mercedes stared ahead and slowly shook her head. After the doctor left, Mercedes began to cry softly. After some time, she spoke, her voice faint and strained. She seemed to be speaking mostly to herself.

"I have so many questions," she said, "but none of them you can answer. Why did this happen to me? Am I being punished? Is this God's response to what I've done?"

Katia clasped Mercedes's hand. She didn't know what to say.

"How long have I been here, Katia? The señora, does she know?"

"I told her you're in the hospital with appendicitis," replied Katia. "Your mother came to Lima to fill in for you until you can return to work."

Mercedes looked up at her with horror and disbelief.

Katia shook her head. "Your mother doesn't know what happened, Mercedes," said Katia. "But she will be coming here soon. She wants to see you."

Mercedes closed her eyes tightly, as if to shut out the world and make it all disappear. Katia tried to think of something reassuring to say, but before she could, Mercedes had drifted off to sleep.

Mercedes steadily got better and after several days was able to leave the hospital. Katia came to pick her up and they sat outside of the hospital at a nearby park, sharing a small lunch.

"Did you know," Mercedes said, "that the whole section of the hospital I was in is for women who've had abortions? The doctor said that women almost die all the time from complications like mine."

"Dios mío!" said Katia. "I didn't realize that it could be so dangerous. You always hear about this or that woman getting one done and then, poof, problem solved! My cousin's friend went to that same man that we visited and was perfectly fine afterward. Well, my cousin said that she was sore and bled a little, but she didn't end up in the hospital."

"Nobody wants to talk about it. That's why abortion is a *secreto de voces* [open secret], something that everyone knows but nobody speaks of. We all know someone who has had an abortion even though it is illegal. People say that it is wrong. But what choice did I have? What choice do any of us have? Our circumstances make the decision, not us." Mercedes sighed. "Everyone is afraid. Afraid that our neighbors, our friends, our priests will condemn us. But women are dying! This wouldn't happen if we could go to real doctors who know how to do things right. This law is killing us."

Katia shook her head. "I remember the days of my youth," she said, "when everything seemed so black and white. But that's not how it really is. It's never an easy decision; nobody wants to have an abortion. And to have to deal with these outcomes—it's terrible."

"If only they knew," reflected Mercedes, "that before we even made the decision, our hearts were already breaking."

They sat in silence for a while and then packed up their things and prepared to go.

"So what can we do?" asked Katia.

"I'm going to tell my story," Mercedes replied. "I don't want other women to go through what I did. In school I was only told not to have sex. I never went to the clinic because I thought that they would think I was a loose woman without values or morals because I didn't have a husband. I felt like there was no other choice for the pregnancy but to end it. I felt so alone, but these things happen to so many women all the time. But if we don't talk about it, if we don't share, then nothing will ever change."

"Who will you tell?" asked Katia.

"At the hospital, they told me about an organization not far from here where women can go to get information and support. This organization also sends people out into the community to talk to girls and women about their health and sexuality and to share their own experiences. I think that I will start there. Even if I can only volunteer on my days off, it will be something. I think that it will help me to recover too. Not in my body, but in my heart and mind. The guilt, the sadness, the anger may never completely go away. But like the physical scars, these emotional ones will fade."

Mercedes smiled at Katia for the first time since she'd been in the hospital. Katia knew that this would be a long journey, but an important one for Mercedes—one to heal her broken heart and to undo the silence of a secret. She felt ready to help her in any way she could. A sad story would be even more tragic if it were never told, especially when it could cultivate seeds of change and hope for a better future.

26
There Will Always Be More Struggles to Win

Lesley Jo Weaver and David Meek

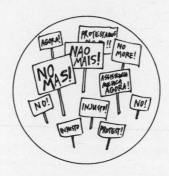

"There Will Always Be More Struggles to Win" is about João Pedro, an eleven-year-old boy who lives in a farming community in rural Brazil. He accompanies his mom, a community health worker, on her visits to local households. By observing what she does and says and thinking about his own experiences, João Pedro learns about how important it is to have access to health care in their isolated village. Health is considered a basic human right under the Universal Declaration of Human Rights, a document created by the United Nations after World War II. As part of this recognition, access to the means of health—that is, to health care—is also considered a human right, but it is still lacking in many parts of the world, especially in rural areas of developing countries in Africa, Latin America, and South Asia. This story illustrates how access to health care is often tied to politics and may not be consistent for many poor people.

João Pedro awoke early to a symphony of rooster calls echoing between his family's farm and the others that surrounded their land. Rocking himself back and forth in his low-slung hammock, he stretched and rubbed the sleepiness out of his eyes. Today was a going-out day. He would put on his cowboy boots and pants and his button-up shirt and sit in front of his mother on the family motorcycle. He swung out of his hammock with excitement, anticipating the wonderful feeling of the wind rippling through his thick dark hair and tickling his ears as they drove down the hilly dirt roads of the farming settlement where they lived in the rural Brazilian Amazon.

Three times a week, João Pedro's mother made house-to-house visits, distributing vitamins, weighing and measuring children, and talking with families about children's health and safety. She and five other women were employed as community health workers by Brazil's government, and each one was responsible for visiting one hundred households each month. João Pedro loved going out to visit the families and play with friends who lived in the houses they would visit, but most of all, he loved watching his mom at work. She was proud of the contribution she was making to the health of their community, and so was João. Only once in a while did João Pedro get to go with her, and today was one of those special days.

"*Vem cá*, João Pedro," called his mom, interrupting his thoughts. "Your breakfast is ready!" Pulling on his second boot, João came running out to the verandah, where a steaming hot bowl of milky *cuzcuz* (cornmeal cereal) awaited him on the high wood table, accompanied by a small jelly jar filled just a quarter of the way with black, sweet coffee. As he began to eat, his mom came onto the porch wearing her blue and white Brazilian Health Service T-shirt and a matching baseball cap. He could still remember the day she came home from her training course with this uniform, and how she smiled proudly when she explained to him that this meant she was now eligible to work in their own community, helping to keep children like him healthy.

The settlement where they lived was founded by a big group of poor people, including João Pedro's grandparents, who wanted to farm but had no land on which to do so. Joining in the huge national movement called Movimento dos Trabalhadores Rurais Sem Terra (Landless Workers' Movement), this group of people had pressured the government to take unused land and create homes for those like his family, who had no land.

About fifteen years earlier, before João Pedro was born, their settlement had won a huge piece of land, and the government helped them arrange it, with plots divided up for each household and a town in the center. Most people in their community were still farmers or cattle ranchers, and although most had a house in the central town area, many, including João Pedro's family, lived part-time or full-time on their farmland outside of town. This flexibility was wonderful, João thought, because it meant that they could visit people in town when they wanted to but could always return to the peace of the countryside when they wanted. In the farmlands, the houses were spaced far apart, and people were sometimes hard to find. That's why the government hired his mom instead of someone from outside their community to work as a health worker. She knew all of the families she visited, and she knew how to find them if they were not at their usual home. Some of the people they were going to visit today were even members of João's own family. In a community of this size, of about six hundred families, almost everyone knew each other.

A few years ago, João Pedro remembered a string of meetings and events that were like parties, which his mother told him were protests. People in the community were demanding the state government build a health center in their own town because when people got sick, they had nowhere nearby to go. The nearest health center at the time was an hour-long drive down a bumpy dirt road, and few people had cars, although many had motorbikes. It was a terrible and difficult thing to take that ride when one was very sick, he knew. If a car could not be located for someone too ill to ride the motorbike, they sometimes simply could not go. He remembered the people at this protest chanting over and over again that health care was a right for all people, not just a privilege for the wealthy. Then one day, people were excited from all ends of the community, shouting that they'd won!

Soon afterward, João Pedro had watched, fascinated as a new structure was built for the health facility. Bricks were stacked and stuccoed
to make the walls, the corrugated tin roof was put on, and the cement
was poured and smoothed for the floors. This was where his mom's new
office would be, so he was interested in what they were building.

The process took over two years, but the community began using
parts of it long before the building was finished. About a year ago, a doctor began coming from the city two mornings a week to see patients in
their community, and finally, a few months ago, the health post was finished and the mayor from the city came for a dedication ceremony. João
Pedro's mom and her five colleagues, who were all community health
workers, now met there to talk about their work every week, and there
was a nurse, a pharmacist, and a man who gave injections to all the children on a special day each month.

Soon it was time to go. After slinging her backpack over her shoulders, João Pedro's mom lifted him onto the motorcycle in front of her
and they drove off, João Pedro holding onto the handlebars tightly and
giggling with delight. Their first stop would be Seu Francisco's house a
few miles away. Although it was only nine o'clock in the morning, the
dry-season sun baked down on them as they kicked up a trail of dust
along the road. This is so different from the wet season, thought João
Pedro. Sometimes these roads get so muddy that we can't even drive
them, but look at them now—they're as hard and dry as a clay pot. They
drove out of their own land plot, over the bridge to the main road, and
away to Seu Francisco's farm.

João Pedro had been looking forward to this visit because he heard
that Seu Francisco's daughter, Rosa, had had a new baby. Like most people in this community, João delighted in playing with little babies, and
now he was getting old enough that he was sometimes even allowed to
hold them. He remembered watching Rosa's belly grow more and more
with each monthly visit, and how his mom would give her special vitamins for pregnancy, to "keep the mom and baby healthy," she said.

Usually babies were born at home in this community, but sometimes
the moms or the babies had difficulties after the birth and had to travel to

the city to stay in the hospital. Just last year, he had gone with his family to a baby's funeral. It made him sad to see the tiny coffin.

Helping moms and babies to be healthy was one of João's mom's most important jobs, and lately she had been trying to encourage women to have their babies in a hospital, even if there was nothing wrong. She said that like the one whose funeral they went to, so many babies had died due to complications after labor because the long journey made it impossible for them to get the medical care they needed in time. Since João's mom and the other health-care workers had begun urging women to give birth outside the settlement, some women had been going to stay with relatives in the town before they started labor. He was anxious to see if this baby was healthy, and he crossed his fingers superstitiously as he thought about it.

The motorcycle pulled up to Seu Francisco's farmhouse with a roar that made the chickens and guinea fowl scatter with indignant clucks. His mom clapped three times to announce their presence outside the open door of the house, and Seu Francisco's wife came bustling out of the kitchen, wiping her hands on a towel. "Entra! Se senta!" she exclaimed, gesturing welcomingly toward the sofa in their front room.

"Will you have some coffee?"

João Pedro's mom never said no to coffee. Soon the customary jelly jar appeared with a little coffee in the bottom.

"Dona Olinda, where is the baby?" asked João Pedro eagerly, no longer able to wait.

"Ah, menino, the baby is not home yet. Rosa went to have her in the hospital, like your mom suggested. But they are doing fine, Rosa and the baby. She was just born yesterday! Here, look at this," she said, pulling out a cell phone and showing a picture of a tiny, dark-haired baby curled in the arms of a tired-looking but smiling Rosa. "They'll be home tomorrow," said Dona Olinda.

"Gracias a Deus," said João Pedro's mom with a sigh of relief. "Congratulations, Dona Olinda! Isn't she cute, João?" she said, smiling. He nodded, staring solemnly at the picture and feeling relieved too. "I'll weigh and measure her next month when I visit," continued his mom.

"Make sure Rosa keeps the baby's health booklet in a safe place, because I'll also need to check her vaccines." Everyone got a health booklet when they were born in Brazil. João Pedro had one, too, with his name on it. It had all kinds of information about João's birth, his height and weight, and his vaccines.

"And how is Seu Francisco?" asked João Pedro's mom. "Is he taking his medicines and watching his diet?" Seu Francisco had diabetes, João knew, which meant he should not have sweets, colas, or too much rice. "Yes," replied Dona Olinda, "he was just at the health post yesterday. He went to get to get a checkup with the doctor. You know, he goes every month to get his medicines. It's so much easier now that the health center is right here. There are still long lines, but it doesn't take all day like it used to when we had to go to the city. Plus, he gets his medicines for free."

This, João Pedro knew, was a big benefit of having the health center in town. He, too, had benefitted from it. Last time João Pedro was sick with a fever, his mom took him there and the doctor gave him antibiotics. This was so much better than taking the hour-long ride through the countryside to town when he was sick, like he used to do.

Soon it was time to go. Their next stop would be Tío (Uncle) Maneu's house. João Pedro loved going there. Tío Maneu, his grandma's brother, grew and sold fruit and vegetables in their town, and his wife, Maria, made fruit-flavored *geladinhos* (ice cream bars) to sell. She almost always gave him one when they went there for a visit, and he would get to play with their grandson, Rodrigo. Rodrigo lived with his grandparents because his parents wanted him to have the opportunity to grow up in the country, like they did before they moved to the city for work. As they pulled up to the house under a big mango tree, João Pedro clapped his hands three times and called, "Hey, Tía Maria! Can we come in? Hey Rodrigo!"

As João and Rodrigo scampered around together, João Pedro's mom got a scale and a pencil out of her backpack. She asked Rodrigo to come over and stand still on the scale, which he could hardly bear to do because he was so excited to see João. Tía Maria produced Rodrigo's health booklet, and João Pedro's mom noted his weight on a chart that showed whether his weight was normal for his age, while Rodrigo fidgeted. "Good," she said. Rodrigo stood up straight against a wall, and João Pedro's mom marked where the top of his head hit the wall with the pencil. Then she turned the page of his health booklet and noted his height on a chart that showed whether his height was normal for his age. "That's good too."

She asked him to look up and pulled down his lower eyelids to check the color of their inside rims in case he might be anemic. Then she turned to the back of the booklet where Rodrigo's vaccine records were. "Hmm, Rodrigo needs a *meningo* [meningitis] vaccine," she observed. "This month's vaccine camp will be next Friday morning in the town square. Bring him then, and we'll make sure it gets done, OK?" Tía Maria nodded. With that, it was time for them to go. João would have liked to stay and play all day, but they had many more houses to visit, so they couldn't stay too long.

João Pedro licked the last of the geladinho from his mouth as they waved good-bye and headed to their next house visit. This was Seu Haroldo's place. Like most of the men in the community, Seu Haroldo was not home during the day. He worked in the town's information center, but his wife and three teenage sons were there.

As they pulled up to the house, João Pedro remembered when he once asked why they had only sons and no daughters. Seu Haroldo became very sad. "We did have one daughter," he explained, "but she choked on a cashew nut and died when she was very young. Being as far out in the countryside as we live, there was nothing we could do— no emergency services to go to, and no one in town with the training to help." As it turned out, this was a common story among people older than João Pedro. His mom, for example, lost two siblings as children to fevers. Tía Maria lost a child too. Only in the last ten years or so had parents stopped losing children in this community. "Maybe," Joao Pedro thought with pride as they rode home at the end of the day, "my mom is helping save some of those kids."

A few weeks later, everyone began preparing for another big party, which João Pedro's mom explained was for the local election, just like the one they had had a few years ago when the health post project had begun. The whole family went one night to a *churrasco* (barbecue) and stuffed themselves on beef and spicy *farinha* (manioc meal) as men gave speeches on a stage. Soon after that, João Pedro's mom came home one day from her work at the health post and seemed very upset. She almost never got sad or angry, so João noticed. "What's wrong, Mom?" he asked hesitantly.

"There won't be doctors coming to the clinic anymore, and my job is getting cut out. It's because of the elections."

"But that big party in town!" João Pedro exclaimed, confused. "I thought people said we won."

Sighing, João's mom explained that they did win the local election, but that there was another big party for the state-level election where they decided to take away the money that was paying the doctor to visit the health post. She explained that they decided no one could afford to hire a doctor to come all the way out to their settlement, and besides, they shouldn't have to pay for a service that the government provided to most Brazilians for free just because they lived where they did. "Even though we won our land, there will always be more struggles to win," she said.

BRAC
Kathy Wollner

BRAC was founded in Bangladesh in 1972 as the Bangladesh Rehabilitation Assistance Committee. The organization, known by its acronym, started its work with relief efforts after the end of the Bangladesh Liberation War, which led to East Pakistan (now Bangladesh) separating from West Pakistan (now Pakistan). The organization's work then focused on the needs of refugees returning from India to northeastern Bangladesh. The next year, 1973, BRAC's work moved away from relief and more toward long-term efforts to improve life in communities, known as *community development*. To show this change in focus, BRAC was renamed the Bangladesh Rural Advancement Committee.

Today BRAC's vision is to create "a world free from all forms of exploitation and discrimination where everyone has the opportunity to realize their potential."[*] Its mission is to "empower people and communities in situations of poverty, illiteracy, disease and social injustice."[†] Both in Bangladesh and globally, BRAC is seen as a pioneer in working to combat poverty through community-level intervention.

BRAC works on many different issues to reduce poverty and help communities but has always focused on health. In Bangladesh, access to health care, especially in rural communities, is poor. As we learned in "There Will Always Be More Struggles to Win," community health workers are very important in educating and treating people in their communities, especially in rural areas. The people who work with BRAC are a part of the communities in which they work. BRAC's

---

[*] "Who We Are: Mission and Vision," BRAC, accessed May 19, 2013, http://www.brac.net/content/who-we-are-mission-vision#.U9bkl8Jow5s.

[†] Ibid.

health program uses a door-to-door approach, with community health workers connecting directly with people who need health services. At current count, 95,623 *shasthya shebikas* (health volunteers) and 10,008 *shasthya karmis* (community health workers) across Bangladesh work to connect people living in rural areas with the formal health system of government and private clinics and hospitals. These volunteers and workers visit people in their homes, so people don't have to depend only on clinics and hospitals for health knowledge and care. This is an important part of the program because many people cannot afford to travel the distance, sometimes many days on foot, to the closest health post or hospital.

Over the past forty-one years, BRAC has overseen many projects that have improved health and health access in Bangladesh. In the 1980s, its Oral Rehydration Therapy Extension Program reached thirteen million households. This program was groundbreaking because it found a simple formula of salt, sugar, and water could reduce child death substantially. It provided a cost-effective formula for fighting diarrhea-related dehydration, a major cause of death for children under five. At the same time, BRAC started a program for directly observed treatment (DOT) for tuberculosis. DOT requires community health workers to observe patients taking their medicines every day to make sure they get the full treatment for their tuberculosis infection. If patients do not complete their treatment, often because they are feeling better, then there is an increased risk of reinfection with more dangerous strains of tuberculosis. With DOT, the patient gets better and there is less tuberculosis in the community. More recently, in the 2000s, BRAC created birthing huts, places for women to give birth in urban slums or very poor areas of cities. These birthing huts have health services available for women and are culturally accepted, meaning they work within the cultural traditions around childbirth in Bangladesh.

Today, BRAC works in seventy thousand villages and two thousand slums, and reaches three-quarters of the Bangladeshi population. It is now the largest development organization in the world, working throughout Asia and Africa as well as in Bangladesh.

DISCUSSION QUESTIONS

- Name two situations in which relief work would make the most sense for a community. Describe another situation in which community development would be best.

- Why is access to health care a challenge in rural areas? Explain one way you've learned about how to improve access to health care in rural communities.

- Access to health care includes access to information, treatment, and health services. Name an example of how BRAC has improved health-care access in Bangladesh in each of these categories.

- Do you know of any organizations in your community that are working to improve health-care access?

- Identify ways that health-care access could be improved in your community.

This section's information has been adapted from BRAC's website. To learn more about BRAC and to see how you can get involved, visit BRAC's website at www.brac.net.

Postscript

Emily Mendenhall

We hope these stories have sparked your curiosity about health in your community and around the world. At its most basic level, we intend for this book to cultivate interest in how the places in which we live and things we experience within those spaces influence our health. For example, how do social relationships influence our health? In what ways can sexual and reproductive health decisions influence mental and physical well-being? How do we cope with mental illness? How does violence influence people's health directly and indirectly? What is the role of prevention in keeping individuals and communities healthy? How can access to health care transform community health in rural and urban areas? These are only some of the questions we hope this book has brought to your attention.

The stories in this book show the complexities of community health, from Tibet to Texas. "Seeking SUCCESS," "The Big Fat Truth," "Dadi's Chart," "Mai'suka, My Island," and "Thiago and the Beach" brought to light how social relationships in people's lives can influence their mental and physical health. Fundamental social and cultural issues around gender and sexuality, which can profoundly affect people's health, were explored in "Slow Motion," "Nditai's Initiation," "Chris Not Christina," "Ariana's Decision," and "My Body, My Self." In "The Ties that Bind," "Chantalle's Secret," "A Homecoming," and "Tenzin's Dream," we explored mental health issues, from recently returned military veterans in the United States to Tibetans exiled to India. We also examined how violence can influence people's lives and impact their health through "Paris of the West," "We All Fight," "Nelson's Soweto," and

"The Grove." This section focused on both interpersonal violence, such as sexual abuse and handgun use, and structural violence, such as the repercussions of poverty on people's health. "Gone Goes the Worm," "A Pandemic Pig Tale," "Route 100," and "Girl Parts" underscored the important role of prevention, through programs and community-wide campaigns, in maintaining community health, from South Sudan to Mexico. Finally, we examined the role of health-care access in keeping people healthy and brought the concepts of accessibility, availability, and affordability of quality health care to the forefront in "Scars," "Mandy and the Motorized Wheelchair," "Open Secrets and Breaking Hearts," and "There Will Always Be More Struggles to Win."

The communites-in-action sections demonstrate how others are transforming community health by working in partnership with communities. The Gay-Straight Alliance Network demonstrates how people with different sexual orientations and gender identities and their allies can come together to empower one another and stand up for equality within their schools. The Texas Freedom Network illustrates the importance of health education and calling for policies that ensure all young people have access to sex education based on science. Sangath stands as an example of an organization working in communities to improve the lives of people with mental illness through the combined efforts of research, programming, and policy. Cure Violence attends to the problem of violence like it is an infectious disease, something that needs to be immediately identified and quarantined in the community. The Sabin Vaccine Institute demonstrates how science can be fundamental to improving health equity. Finally, BRAC is an exemplary organization that works to promote health through low-cost interventions and community-empowerment efforts among some of the world's poorest communities.

By no means do the narratives or examples of community action in this book represent all the issues that affect communities and the health of the people who inhabit them. After reading this book, we hope that you have become curious about learning more about how the places we live, people we interact with, and ways we cope with difficult situations can shape people's health. And we hope that this curiosity is funneled into improving your community in some way.

We have brought to light some of the ways you can identify needs in your communities and take action to change things that may cause harm. We hope that you will bring this information into your lives, be it as an active community member or as a future health-care professional. We hope you use it to help improve the health of your family and the people around you. Community health is an important but complex concept that requires people to understand the many dimensions of what keeps individuals, villages, cities, and nations healthy. It takes many devoted people to contribute to making sure that people can live the healthiest and most fulfilling lives possible, for themselves, their families, and their communities.

A key component of making a difference is understanding the problem. We hope this book has ignited your interest to explore how the places we live and people we interact with can shape our health. To learn more, visit our website (Global Health Narratives for Change, www. GHN4C.org), where we have supplemental educational materials, additional references for more in-depth study of community health, materials for community action, and contacts for organizations working in the field.

Teaching Guide

Kathy Wollner

HOW TO USE THIS GUIDE

This guide has been created to assist teachers who wish to incorporate *Community Health Narratives* into their health, environmental studies, or mainstream education curriculum. We have developed it as a supplement to existing curricula for students in middle school or high school.

Each of the sections below will explain the information found in the content: objectives, guiding questions, prerequisite knowledge, discussion questions, and additional activity options.

Objectives

For each session, there will be distinct objectives according to content. In general, the inclusion of the narratives is for interdisciplinary purposes. The narratives benefit many different fields of study across age and subject matter. Health instruction serves to facilitate discussion and create a framework through which students can understand these important health topics. The inclusion of narratives in social studies, English, and environmental science instruction assists students in making connections among society, politics, economy, and environment and the health challenges people face around the world.

Narratives can either be read aloud during class time while students follow along in their books or read by students independently prior to the lesson. Teaching these narratives may serve as an independent unit or in conjunction with other units to enhance their meaning to the students.

Guiding Questions

Guiding questions will be provided for each topic or narrative. Instructors may prompt students to journal on these questions for approximately ten minutes. Students may write at least three to four sentences in response to the questions. Instructors may alternately ask students to simply keep these overarching questions in mind while they study the narratives related to this topic and cross-curricular connections.

Prerequisite Knowledge

One or more questions will be posed that address prerequisite knowledge for reading a particular narrative. Instructors will go over these questions, provide key definitions prior to reading the narratives, and encourage students to mark any other words or concepts they do not understand as they read along with the narratives. Instructors may use a KWL (what students "Know—Want to Know—Learned") graphic organizer or chart with students throughout the process.

Discussion Questions

Several questions will be provided for instructors as examples of what can be explored during class discussion. Instructors are encouraged to add additional questions that are related to educational standards and/or pertinent to making connections between the narratives and the standard curriculum.

These questions can be utilized in various ways:

1. As the basis of an introduction or "hook" activity. Ideas from these stories may be used to incite conversation at the beginning of a class unit.

2. Incorporated into an open, full-classroom discussion.

3. Used to facilitate small-group discussions. For example, each small group could be assigned one or two questions to discuss, answer in written form, and present to their classmates.

4. As the basis of a wraparound activity. For this activity, each question is written on a sheet of butcher paper. These sheets of butcher paper are then posted around the classroom. Students take turns contributing answers to these questions; each student should contribute at least one unique answer to each question. Students will then volunteer to present two to three answers from each piece of paper. Students do not have to present their own idea but can read and explain an answer contributed by a classmate.

Additional Activity Options

Suggested activities that can be used after the discussion of the narratives will be provided. These activities are meant to supplement the narratives in illustrating the concepts of each lesson. These may include visual or audio aids, journal prompts, or other assignments.

SOCIAL TIES

Social ties are intrinsic to many aspects of our lives: where we live, where and how we learn, what we do for work, what we eat, how we spend our time, and the types of experiences we encounter every day. Social ties affect a person's ability not only to cope with disease but also to maintain a healthy life. This lesson will address the role that family, school, the health-care system, and the broader community play in disease management and health maintenance.

In "Dadi's Chart," students will learn about the challenges of chronic-disease management and how family support can help. In "Seeking success," students will explore the impact of education and family support—or lack thereof—in developing health literacy and gaining the tools needed to advance in life.

Objectives

- Explain how education and health are connected.
- Name the supportive people in Taylor's and Dadi's lives.

- Identify characteristics of individuals and communities that make them supportive.
- Describe the role of social support in managing a chronic disease like diabetes.

Guiding Questions

How do the people around us affect our health? What does it mean to manage a disease? What influence does social support have in making positive changes (e.g., eating healthy, quitting smoking)?

Dadi's Chart

PREREQUISITE KNOWLEDGE

Students should be familiar with the following terms:

Caste. A social class one is born into; Hindu tradition in India.

Imported. Brought to one country from another country.

DISCUSSION QUESTIONS

- What motivated Anjali to make the chart for Dadi?
- What changes do people with diabetes have to make in their lifestyles?
- How does diabetes affect the body long term?
- What are some challenges people face when trying to eat healthy and exercise?
- If you were Dadi, how would you feel about having your grand-daughter be your health helper?

Seeking success

PREREQUISITE KNOWLEDGE

Students should be familiar with the following terms:

Charter school. Whereas the public school a student attends is based on where he or she lives, a charter school is a school that is not publicly run and at which students must be accepted in order to attend. Often, so many students wish to attend that there are lotteries for acceptance. SUCCESS Academy is an example of a charter school.

DISCUSSION QUESTIONS

- Why is Taylor upset with Ms. Hamlin at the beginning of the story?

- How do health problems affect Taylor's life?

- Why can't Taylor read? What could have gone differently for her before she got to fourth grade unable to do her homework?

- Who in Taylor's life supports her? Who does she see as holding her back?

- Do you think Taylor can be successful in life, even if she isn't able to attend SUCCESS Academy?

ADDITIONAL ACTIVITY OPTIONS

- *Develop a health-helper plan.* Each student should identify a person in his or her life who is living with a chronic disease. Examples of chronic diseases include diabetes, high blood pressure, heart failure, asthma, depression, and HIV. If unable to identify someone, students can create a hypothetical person for whom they will serve as a health helper. Students should prepare a plan for how they would be a health helper to that person, as Anjali was in developing a chart for Dadi. Time should be allotted for researching the disease they will address (recommended resource: www.familydoctor.org). If students have trouble identifying specific ways they would help manage the disease, they can include in their plan how they aim to learn more.

- *Watch* Waiting for Superman and *discuss as a class. Waiting for Superman* is a controversial film about the U.S. public school system and the role charter schools may play in changing educational opportunities for inner-city students. One critical review of the documentary, "Grading 'Waiting for Superman'" by Dana Goldstein, appeared in the *Nation* (available online). After reading excerpts of this review, students can develop their own critique of the film or of the education system given the additional information presented in this review. This activity is more appropriate for advanced students.

GENDER AND SEXUALITY

Gender and sexuality are often difficult subjects to broach in the classroom, but they are universal to the human experience. Adolescence is a time when most students begin to have questions about these issues, and using these narratives to incorporate the information about puberty, sexual initiation, pregnancy, and sexually transmitted infection (STI) prevention into a health curriculum can help students to critically consider these issues in a lesson format that focuses on these characters instead of on themselves.

In "Slow Motion," students will learn about puberty through the eyes of Matt, a young man who is frustrated he is not developing as quickly as his peers. This story would be especially helpful if it is integrated into a middle school curriculum. In "Ariana's Decision," students learn about a variety of issues, including romantic attraction, sexual initiation, and pregnancy options. These challenging topics are essential to young people's education. Contrary to common belief, information about sex does not promote sexual activity among young people; it simply gives them the tools they need to prevent unwanted pregnancy and infection when they do choose to have sex, either in adolescence or later in life.

Objectives

- Name three changes that typically occur during puberty.
- Explain how puberty is different for girls and boys.

- Identify the factors a person should consider when deciding whether to have sex.

- Describe the challenges that Ariana faces once she becomes pregnant.

- Name at least two types of birth control and describe the three pregnancy options.

Guiding Questions

What are the changes our bodies undergo during puberty? How do these changes affect us? How do we decide when to have sex? How might a pregnancy change a person's life?

Slow Motion

PREREQUISITE KNOWLEDGE

Students should be familiar with the following terms:

Puberty. The time in life when a person becomes sexually mature. It involves physical changes that usually happen between ages ten and fourteen for girls and ages twelve and sixteen for boys.

Hormones. The body's chemical messengers, which affect growth and development, metabolism (how the body gets energy from food), sexual function, reproduction, and mood. If puberty is truly delayed (no sign of puberty by fourteen for girls or by sixteen for boys), exogenous hormones, or hormones that are made in a lab instead of naturally by the human body, can be given by a doctor if indicated, in an attempt to start puberty.

DISCUSSION QUESTIONS

- Why do you think Matt is concerned about being short, "scrawny," and hairless?

- Do you think Matt's dad is concerned for the same reasons? Why or why not?

- Dr. Brenner asks Matt's dad to leave the room so he can talk to Matt alone. Has your doctor ever done this when you've had a checkup? If so, how did it feel? If not, would you like him or her to do this in the future?

- Why do you think Matt decided to quit basketball?

- When Matt turned fifteen, what changes did his body undergo due to puberty?

Ariana's Decision

PREREQUISITE KNOWLEDGE
Students should be familiar with the following terms:

Unintended pregnancy. When a woman becomes pregnant when she had not planned or intended to become pregnant, meaning the pregnancy is either mistimed or not wanted. In the United States, about half (49 percent) of pregnancies are unintended.

Birth control. There are many types of birth control, or ways to prevent pregnancy. They include condoms, pills, injections, patches, rings, intrauterine devices, and implants. Pregnancy can also be prevented by choosing not to have sex, often called abstinence. Students should learn about these different birth-control options as part of this lesson (recommended resources: www.plannedparenthood.org or www.womenhealth.gov).

DISCUSSION QUESTIONS
- What are the first signs Ariana gets that she may be pregnant?

- Name three factors that played into Ariana's decision to have sex with Chris. If Ariana was your friend, and you knew she was going to the party, what would you tell or ask her?

- Name three ways to prevent pregnancy. What type of birth control also prevents sexually transmitted infections?

- What three options for pregnancy does Dr. Hernandez explain to

Ariana? If you were Ariana, what questions would you have for the doctor?

- *Find out more about puberty.* Students can spend time with the BBC's interactive body, an interface where students can click on certain parts of the body to learn about the changes that take place there. (See www.bbc.co.uk/science/humanbody/body/interactives/lifecycle/teenagers/.)

- *Check sexual health knowledge with a quiz game.* SexualityandU.ca, created by the Society of Obstetricians and Gynecologists of Canada, features information on puberty, contraception, STI prevention, and sexual well-being with a comprehensive, positive approach to sexuality. SexFu Challenge (under Games and Apps) takes students through a series of questions on the male and female reproductive systems, contraception, STIs, and healthy sexuality and self-esteem. Each true or false question shows the correct answer with a thorough explanation. Have students write out the answers to the questions they answered incorrectly to reinforce knowledge. Also, have them write down any further questions they may have, which can be placed in an anonymous question box. The instructor can then review answers to these questions during the next lesson.

MENTAL ILLNESS

Mental illness affects many people worldwide but is, unfortunately, stigmatized in many communities. Just like physical illnesses, mental illnesses can be managed with the right treatment, care, and support. Mental illnesses are caused by an imbalance of neurotransmitters, which are chemicals within the brain that affect our mood, our emotions, and our reactions to experiences. This is a biological cause. Life experiences, however, also play strongly into mental health or illness. As a teacher, you can expand your knowledge on youth mental health through independent teacher training at www.teenmentalheath.org.

In "A Homecoming," Luke's family teaches us about post–traumatic stress disorder and how Luke's father's illness stems from his experiences as a soldier in wartime. In "Chantalle's Secret," Chantalle's circumstances—her poverty and dependence on her in-laws—play into her depression and her attempted suicide. These stories introduce students to common mental health problems and challenge them to think of mental illnesses just as they think of asthma or high blood pressure, as health problems that can improve with treatment and are deserving of attention.

Objectives

- Define post-traumatic stress disorder (PTSD). Identify Luke's dad's actions related to his PTSD.

- Explain the treatments available for people struggling with mental illness.

- Identify ways to prevent suicide.

- Describe the role of support from family or friends for individuals living with mental illness.

Guiding Questions

Are mental illnesses different from other illnesses? Why do people often go through mental illness alone? How can we better take care of mental illness in our communities?

A Homecoming

PREREQUISITE KNOWLEDGE
Students should be familiar with the following terms:

Iraq War. The United States invaded Iraq in March 2003, over-throwing the government and establishing a new, democratic government. A total of 4,487 Americans were killed in combat and

32,226 were injured. The last U.S. military personnel were withdrawn in December 2011.

Post-traumatic stress disorder (PTSD). A disorder characterized by flashbacks; nightmares; hypervigilance; or being easily startled and irritability. It is common among soldiers who have been to war in Iraq or Afghanistan, with studies estimating at least one in five returning veterans from these wars has PTSD.

DISCUSSION QUESTIONS

- What behaviors does Luke begin to notice that make him worried about his dad?
- Why do you think Luke's dad doesn't want to go to the basketball game?
- What is the turning point for Luke's family that leads to his father getting help?
- How did Luke's dad's symptoms improved after seeing the psychologist?
- What are some other experiences, besides being a soldier, that might cause PTSD?

Chantalle's Secret

PREREQUISITE KNOWLEDGE
Students should be familiar with the following terms:

Depression. A common mental illness characterized by depressed mood; lack of interest in things; hopelessness or guilt; poor sleep, energy, and concentration; psychomotor retardation (making movements more slowly than usual); and suicidal thoughts (thinking about ending your life or thinking the world would be better off without you)

Haiti. A small country that occupies the west side of the island Hispaniola, next to the Dominican Republic. It is the poorest country in the Western Hemisphere and was the location of a devastating earthquake in 2010.

DISCUSSION QUESTIONS

- What are some of the factors contributing to Chantalle's depression?
- Why do you think she feels she has no other choice but to end her life?
- Name some of the reasons the community members give for why Chantalle may have attempted suicide. What do these reasons tell us about how suicide and mental illness are viewed in this community?
- What does Étienne do to help Chantalle?
- How do you think Chantalle's future will play out?

ADDITIONAL ACTIVITY OPTIONS

- *Create a Venn diagram.* Students should compare and contrast Luke's dad's and Chantalle's experiences with mental illness. These questions can be considered in the diagram's creation.

  - How did life experiences influence their mental illnesses?
  - How is mental illness viewed in their communities?
  - Is mental illness common?
  - How did their families react to their distress?
  - What led to them getting help?
  - Who did they turn to for support?

- *Learn about resources for suicide prevention.* Students should research resources available to people who are suicidal or who are trying to get help for a friend or family member. Is there a number to call? What if you see a classmate's post on Facebook that says he wants to end his life or a friend's post on Twitter that says her life is worthless? Students should create a plan for what they would do if they needed emotional support or felt they needed to find help for a friend.

VIOLENCE

Violence takes its toll on both individuals and communities. Unfortunately, violence is pervasive in many communities, and this culture of violence often extends onto school grounds. Violence encompasses both the emotional and the physical—from bullying and discrimination to rape and gunshots. Educating students about violence as a health concern is incredibly important in all communities. Where violence is an epidemic, as it is in Nelson's home community, this teaching is needed to show students that violence is not the only way to solve conflict and to give students an opportunity to process and contextualize their experiences. In communities where violence is less pervasive, it is needed to highlight injustice where it does present itself and to challenge students to ask questions about the differences between their community and another. Structural violence—or underlying inequity in social structures—is at the core of this discussion.

In "Nelson's Soweto," students learn about the impact of gun violence on Nelson's family and on his entire neighborhood. In "Paris of the West," Juliana shows students how sexual abuse as a child can continue to impact a person's life into adolescence and adulthood. Her path to recovery demonstrates important components of wellness for people recovering from trauma.

Objectives

- Identify three factors associated with violence in Soweto and other communities like it.
- Describe how life has changed in South Africa since the end of apartheid and how inequality still exists.
- Name both physical and emotional effects of violence.
- Explain the connection between experiencing violence and mental health problems.

Guiding Questions

How does violence affect individuals and communities? What makes people commit violent acts?

Nelson's Soweto

PREREQUISITE KNOWLEDGE

Students should be familiar with the following terms:

Apartheid. A system of racial segregation and discrimination against nonwhites in South Africa from 1950 to 1991.

HIV and AIDS. Human immunodeficiency virus, HIV, is a virus that is carried in the blood, semen, and vaginal fluids. It can be transmitted through unprotected sex. HIV is the virus that causes acquired immune deficiency syndrome, or AIDS, a disease where the immune system is no longer able to fight infection normally. AIDS is a common cause of death in South Africa.

Stigma. A mark of disgrace related to a particular circumstance, quality, or person. HIV and AIDS are very stigmatized diseases.

DISCUSSION QUESTIONS

- Why do you think Mama Hu didn't speak about Nelson's mother's death?

- Why does Mama Hu put up bars on the windows? What does she think causes the violence in their neighborhood?

- Now that apartheid has ended, does inequality still exist in South Africa? How so?

- How has losing Rhulani affected Nelson and Mama Hu?

- Mama Hu tells Nelson to "be better." What do you think this means? How can he "be better"?

Paris of the West

PREREQUISITE KNOWLEDGE

Students should be familiar with the following terms:

Food desert. An area with little or no access to large grocery stores that offer fresh and affordable foods needed to maintain a healthy diet. Instead of grocery stores, these areas often contain many fast-food restaurants and convenience stores. Juliana describes her home city as a food desert.

DISCUSSION QUESTIONS

• How does where Juliana lives affect her? Is there anything in your community has that Juliana's Detroit lacks?

• At the beginning of the story, how did Juliana view her sexual abuse? Who does she blame?

• How is Mr. Jackson different from Juliana's other teachers? How does he help Juliana?

• What role does Annie play in Juliana's recovery? Why do you think Juliana was able to tell Annie her story?

• How does taking part in the group change the way that Juliana views what happened to her and her outlook on life?

ADDITIONAL ACTIVITY OPTIONS

• The Interrupters *viewing and class discussion. The Interrupters* is a film about the organization Cure Violence, which works to stop the spread of violence in inner cities. Students can also read about this organization in the "Violence" section. Compare and contrast gun violence in Chicago to gun violence in Soweto, Johannesburg.

• *Discuss violence in your community*. Violence exists in all communities. From the emotional abuse of a parent telling a child he or she isn't good enough to gun violence, which may affect behavior throughout a neighborhood. Students can discuss in small groups or write independent reflections pondering the following questions:

- What types of violence are common in your community?
- How does violence change how people live on a daily basis?
- How has violence impacted your life?
- Do you know anyone who has been harmed by violence?
- How could you work to decrease violence in your community?

PREVENTION

Prevention of disease at the individual and community level is essential to community health. Prevention includes vaccinations, sanitation and clean water, healthy eating, exercise, and antismoking and anti–substance use programs. While prevention of communicable or infectious disease can often be straightforward—for example, hepatitis B is prevented by a vaccine given in childhood—it can also be complex, as we learn from Anok in "Gone Goes the Worm." Guinea worm is prevented by changing many behaviors within the community to ensure that water and, therefore, people stay free from guinea worm.

Cancer screening is also prevention in that it prevents atypical cell development from progressing to cancer or finds tumors when they are in their early stages and are more treatable. In "Girl Parts," we learn about screening for cervical cancer, but other cancers can and should be screened for as well. Mammograms screen for breast cancer and colonoscopies screen for colon cancer. Jared's mom's story teaches us some barriers to disease screening and introduces students to the consequences of delaying care for economic reasons.

Objectives
- Explain why it is better to prevent a disease than to treat it later.
- Identify and describe barriers to disease prevention.

- Describe the life cycle of the guinea worm and where the community can intervene to prevent its transmission.

- Name two different ways to prevent cervical cancer. Explain how health-care providers screen or check for this cancer.

- Describe how poor access to health care can impact disease prevention and screening.

Guiding Questions

Why do some diseases occur in some parts of the world but not others? Why must communities all work together to prevent a disease like guinea worm? What does it mean to screen for a disease?

Gone Goes the Worm

PREREQUISITE KNOWLEDGE

Students should be familiar with the following terms:

Life cycle. A period that involves one generation of an organism through reproduction. Anok describes the life cycle of the guinea worm in the story he tells with the cloth flip chart.

DISCUSSION QUESTIONS

- Why does Ngong ask Anok's sister where she gets the water? How does a person get guinea worm?

- Why do you think Anok was named the new village volunteer? Is he good at his job? Why or why not?

- Why does Anok's uncle doubt the story of the guinea worm from the cloth flip chart? How does Anok respond to his doubts?

- What are the community's rules that are put in place with Anok as village volunteer? Are they always followed? How did the rules help prevent guinea worm?

Girl Parts

PREREQUISITE KNOWLEDGE

Students should be familiar with the following terms:

Human papillomavirus (HPV). A virus that is transmitted sexually and through intimate skin-to-skin contact. It can change cells in the cervix, anus, penis, and head/neck to grow in abnormal ways, which can turn into cancer.

Pap smear. A screening test for cervical cancer. It involves the removal of cells from the cervix to look for any abnormality that might be developing into cancer. Cells can also be tested for HPV to see if this virus is present.

DISCUSSION QUESTIONS

- How does Jared respond to his mother's news? Why do you think he reacts this way? What does he do next?

- How can cervical cancer be prevented?

- Why didn't Jared's mom get her pap smear earlier?

- What did Jared learn about HPV and how it relates to him?

- How did Jared's relationship with his mom change over the course of the story?

ADDITIONAL ACTIVITY OPTIONS

- *Find a copy of your own vaccination record*. Choose one of the vaccines listed and research that illness. How did this disease affect children before a vaccine was able to prevent it?

- *Learn more about HPV and other sexually transmitted infections (STIs)*. Students will perform Internet searches to find the following information (recommended resource: MedlinePlus at www.nlm.nih.gov/medlineplus/).

  - Does HPV have any symptoms?

- Besides vaccination and checkups, what are other ways people can protect themselves from HPV and other STIs?

- Besides cervical cancer, are there other types of cancer that are caused by HPV? Do these only affect women?

- Name other common STIs that can be detected by getting yourself tested.

- Does birth control, like pills for example, prevent STIs?

- Is there a cure for HPV?

- According to the most up-to-date information (as of 2013), at what age should women start getting pap smears to screen for cervical cancer?

- *Investigate other ways to screen for cancer.* Students should look up other types of cancer that can be screened for and learn how to screen for them. Students should ask their parents or other family members about cancer screening. Should they be screened based on how old they are? If so, have they been screened? Why or why not?

HEALTH-CARE ACCESS

Health-care access is imperative for preventing, treating, and caring for disease. This can be realized in many different ways and includes components of accessibility, availability, affordability, and quality. Access includes places, such as hospitals or clinics; human resources, such as health-care professionals or community health workers; and tools, such as surgical supplies. It also involves a system of payment for care that is not prohibitive so all people can afford to access health care.

In "Scars," students meet Ronnie, who serves as an advocate for his sick grandfather. Students are challenged to think about the challenges faced by immigrants, specifically refugees, and to grapple with the concept of cultural competence in health care. In "There Will Always Be More Struggles to Win," students are introduced to a system of health-care administration that they may not have seen before, one grounded by the efforts of community health workers. They also have the opportunity to think about the role of political advocacy in improving access to health care and how they might work for health justice in their community.

Objectives

- Explain the role of traditional healing for refugees like Ronnie's mzee.

- Name at least two barriers to health care for refugees or other individuals who immigrate to a new country.

- Describe the challenges Ronnie faces while acting as his mzee's health advocate.

- Define health-care access and identify some barriers to good health-care access.

- Describe the role of community health workers in areas with poor access to health care.

Guiding Questions

How does access to health care influence people's health? How might limited access affect a community? What are some ways to improve access in communities that are rural or have few resources?

Scars

PREREQUISITE KNOWLEDGE
Students should be familiar with the following terms:

Internally displaced person. A person who has to leave his or her homeland and travel away from it but doesn't cross a border out of their home country.

Refugee. A person who has to leave his or her homeland and travel away from it into country different from their home country.

Cultural competence. The ability to interact effectively with people of different cultures and social or economic backgrounds. This is an especially important skill for health-care providers.

DISCUSSION QUESTIONS

- What makes Ronnie and then Justin stand out at their school? How does this make Ronnie feel? How does Ronnie initially distance himself from Justin?

- Why does Ronnie's mzee trust Dr. Okino? Why doesn't he trust the "Western doctors"?

- Identify the two things Ronnie does to convince his mzee to go to this clinic. Which do you think was most effective. Why?

- What ends up being the cause of mzee's cough? How is this disease transmitted from person to person? Is it curable?

- Who are the members of Ronnie's family at the end of the story? What makes them family?

There Will Always Be More Struggles to Win

PREREQUISITE KNOWLEDGE
Students should be familiar with the following terms:

United Nations (UN). An international organization formed in 1945 to bring all nations of the world together to work for peace and development. There are currently 192 nation members in the UN's General Assembly.

Community health worker. A member of the community chosen to provide basic health care and health education to the community. Such a person is different from doctors or nurses, who are called "highly educated health professionals" and are often few and far between in poor countries.

Brazilian Amazon. Sixty percent of the Amazon rain forest is within the country of Brazil in South America. This area of Brazil is very remote and has low population density, meaning there is a lot of space for few people.

- Why is land so important to people in João's settlement?
- How did people get health care before the clinic was built? What changed in the community after the clinic opened? Name some examples.
- What are João's mom's tasks as a community health worker?
- What arguments does the new government make for no longer sending a doctor to the clinic? How could you counter the new government's argument?
- If you were João or his mom, what would you do next?

- *Read the Universal Declaration of Human Rights.* Identify the articles that have to do with health and health care. What do the other articles focus on? Do these parts of the declaration also relate to health in any way?

- *Create a poster.* Join João Pablo's community's next protest! As a member of the settlement, participate in a protest to bring the doctor back to the clinic and reinstate João's mom as a community health worker. Create a poster with a message on it that speaks to access to health care in this community. What would you do to convince other community members to join the protest? Use the message on your poster to convince a classmate to work with you.

- *Learn about the health-care system in the United States.* Examine the issues of accessibility, availability, affordability, and quality in your community. How do they relate to the national health-care system as a whole? Students should respond to questions listed in one of the bullet points below. They should then share what they have learned with their classmates in a brief presentation.

- Who delivers health care? Are hospitals and clinics public (run by the government) or private?

- How is health care paid for? What is health insurance? What kinds of health insurance exist? Do people in your community have trouble affording health care? Do they ever decide not to go to the clinic or hospital because of cost?

- How has politics influenced the health-care system? Have any new laws been passed recently that affect the health-care system?

- Do all people have equal access to the health-care system? Why or why not?

Contributors

Brian Ackerman, MSc, works in advertising sales and communications consulting in Washington, D.C., at the FP Group, publisher of *Foreign Policy* magazine and ForeignPolicy.com. Prior to working at FP, he worked as a researcher at a firm in Washington, D.C., that provides management consulting analysis for higher education institutions. He has also served as a lobbyist on U.S. foreign policy regarding global HIV/AIDS and reproductive health policy for young people. His story was inspired by experiences he had while living in Rio for two years as a Rotary Ambassadorial Scholar during his graduate education in political geography.

Hannah Adams Burque has been drawing small pictures all of her life. She studied studio art at Bard College and runs a music-licensing company (Ghost Town, Inc.) with her husband.

Bechara Choucair, MD, is commissioner of the Chicago Department of Public Health, appointed in 2009 by Mayor Richard M. Daley. He has worked extensively as a physician with vulnerable populations in the United States and Lebanon, where he was born. Bechara has served as medical director of Crusader Community Health in Rockford, Illinois, executive director of Heartland International Health Center, and vice chair of Community Medicine at Northwestern University's Feinberg School of Medicine. He also has received many awards for his service to community health.

Fiona Cresswell, MD, DTM&H, works as a physician in the field of HIV and sexual health in Brighton, England. Fiona is a trustee of Health Improvement Project Zanzibar, which aims to strengthen health systems in Zanzibar, a semiautonomous region of Tanzania. She is on the faculty of the East African Diploma in Tropical Medicine and Hygiene, teaches in an MSc degree program in global health, and teaches medical undergraduates about HIV and sexual and reproductive health.

Erin P. Finley, PhD, MPH, is a medical anthropologist and health services researcher with the South Texas Veterans Health Care System and assistant professor in the Division of Hospital Medicine, Department of Medicine, and the Department of Psychiatry at the University of Texas Health Science Center in San Antonio. Her research focuses on posttraumatic stress disorder among American veterans and their families and on the implementation of evidence-based practices in inpatient and outpatient settings.

Erica Gibson, PhD, is an assistant professor in the Department of Anthropology and the Women's and Gender Studies Program at the University of South Carolina. She is a biocultural medical anthropologist trained in the four-field approach. Her research is centered on reproductive health care among Latina women in Mexico and the United States.

Ashley Hagaman, MPH, is an anthropology and global health PhD student in the School of Human Evolution and Social Change at Arizona State University. Previously, she helped develop a nonprofit called GlobeMed, working to educate and train student advocates for global health equity. Her research focuses on understanding the drivers of suicide and mental distress in low- and middle-income countries.

Lauren Slubowski Keenan-Devlin, PhD, MPH, is a biocultural anthropologist who is passionate about reducing health disparities in Chicago. She has spent the past few years working in schools and community programs on Chicago's West Side, learning about the impacts of neighborhood environments and community empowerment on kids' well-being.

Ember Keighley, MD, MPH, is a family medicine doctor in Northern California, where she works to care for underserved communities. She has worked on public health and medicine projects in Mexico, Samoa, American Samoa, Ghana, and Mongolia and is dedicated to helping improve the health and well-being of people in underserved communities around the world.

Patrick Klacza is a writer, musician, and native Chicagoan. He received his MFAW from the School of the Art Institute of Chicago in 2013. A writer of short stories and novels, Klacza has never had a cavity.

Adam Koon, MPH, is a PhD candidate in the Politics and Policy Group at the London School of Hygiene and Tropical Medicine. Previously he worked as a technical advisor for the Carter Center's guinea worm eradication program in South Sudan. He also has worked in Kenya, India, and South Africa and currently is conducting health policy research in Nairobi. He coedited the second book in this series, *Environmental Health Narratives* (2012).

Stephen Lavenberg is passionate about addressing global health disparities and health and human rights. He recently returned to the United States after living for the past two years in northern Uganda under the auspices of the Peace Corps. The people he met there inspired him to write for this book and to continue striving for his dreams.

Sara Lewis, MSW, PhD, is a visiting assistant professor at the University of Oregon; her research interests lie at the intersections between mental health, culture, and religion. Her dissertation research involved fourteen months of ethnographic fieldwork in Dharamsala, India, investigating how Buddhism and other sociocultural factors support coping and resilience among Tibetan refugees. She has also served as a coinvestigator on research related to mental health and recovery in the United States and has worked as a psychotherapist in community mental health, focusing on the treatment of serious and persistent mental illness.

Judi Marcin, MD, grew up in Florida but currently lives in Chicago. She is a part-time faculty member in family medicine, working to integrate a humanities curriculum into her residency program. Judi is also a candidate in the MFA in Writing for Children and Young Adults program at Hamline University in St. Paul, Minnesota. She believes stories are the heart and soul of our lives and that there is no better way to share them than through writing.

David Meek, PhD, is an instructor in the Department of Anthropology at the University of Alabama. His research focuses on how people learn through political participation, and the potential impact this learning has on agricultural practices and landscape changes. David's dissertation research focused on the relationships between public policies, economic incentives, and educational processes within an agrarian reform settlement in the Brazilian Amazon.

Emily Mendenhall, PhD, MPH, is a medical anthropologist and an assistant professor of global health at Georgetown University's Edmund A. Walsh School of Foreign Service. Her research examines women's health in cities in the United States, India, Kenya, and South Africa. She is committed to developing global health curricula that are engaging for those curious about global health inequalities, such as *Global Health Narratives* (2009) and *Environmental Health Narratives* (2012). She is founding director of the nonprofit organization Global Health Narratives for Change (www.GHN4C.org).

Neely Myers, PhD, is an assistant professor of anthropology at Southern Methodist University. As a critical medical and psychiatric anthropologist, she has conducted research in low-resource settings in the United States and Tanzania on the everyday experiences of people who have experienced psychosis and trauma (war, torture, intimate-partner violence). She founded Global Public Psychiatry, a consortium committed to improving global mental health care. Her first book, *Recovery, Moral Agency, and Mental Health Care: An Ethnography*, is forthcoming in 2015.

Molly O'Brien is a senior at Elon University studying anthropology and creative writing. Her research interests include education and health care for low-income families in North Carolina. She currently lives in Apex, North Carolina, and plans to begin working toward an MFA in creative writing in the fall of 2014.

Chandra Y. Osborn, PhD, MPH, is an assistant professor of medicine and biomedical informatics at Vanderbilt University Medical Center. Her research focuses on improving care for racial/ethnic minorities, identifying modifiable determinants of medication adherence and health disparities, identifying when "the digital divide" may exacerbate disparities, and leveraging technologies to improve patient adherence.

Aunchalee E. L. Palmquist, PhD, IBCLC, is an assistant professor of anthropology at Elon University. She is a medical anthropologist with research interests in infant- and child-feeding beliefs and practices, breastfeeding, and health disparities. She has conducted ethnographic research in Thailand, Palau, Hawaii, and the mainland United States. Currently she is conducting a study of Internet-based milk sharing in the United States.

Kelley Alison Smith, MA, MPH, is a global health project manager, academic editor, and writing instructor. Her work has taken her to South Africa, Kenya, Ethiopia, and Bangladesh. In 2010 she lived in American Samoa managing a diabetes-research project. Her favorite part of being there was the snorkeling. She lives in Rhode Island with her family and often writes about health-care issues.

Suzanne Farrell Smith, MFA, MA, is a writer whose essays, memoir, and stories have been widely published in literary and academic journals, including the *Kenyon Review*, the *Writer's Chronicle*, *Post Road*, *PANK*, the *Monarch Review*, and the *English Record*. Much of her work combines neuroscience, psychology, and memoir. She has been teaching for fifteen years, most recently as a college writing instructor. Suzanne lives with her husband and son at the foot of the United Nations in Midtown Manhattan.

Charlie Speicher, MA, is a school counselor at an alternative high school in Browning, Montana. He has long been passionate about issues in Indian Country and works extensively with Native American adolescents struggling with grief and loss. He and his wife live in East Glacier in the shadow of the Rocky Mountains. Charlie also loves death metal and climbing mountains.

Lesley Jo Weaver, PhD, MPH, is an assistant professor of anthropology at the University of Alabama. She is a medical anthropologist who focuses on the complex relationships between economic development, changing social roles, mental health, and the everyday management of chronic illnesses like type 2 diabetes. She has conducted research on type 2 diabetes and mental health in India, as well as on food insecurity and mental health in Brazil.

Kathy Wollner, MD, is a family medicine resident physician in Seattle, Washington. She has worked with GHN4C for the past three years and developed teaching guides for *Global Health Narratives* (2009) and *Environmental Health Narratives* (2012) based on her work with the Student Health Force in Chicago. She has learned, worked, and explored in communities in the United States, Chile, and Kenya.

Heather Wurtz, BSN, is a PhD student in medical anthropology and a fellow in the Gender, Sexuality, and Health Training Program at Columbia University. She has worked as a registered nurse in obstetrics and has conducted ethnographic research on women's reproductive and sexual health in the United States, Peru, and Ecuador. Heather's current research focuses on reproductive politics, health-care access, and transnational migration among Mexican-origin women in southern Texas.

Index

abortion, 88, 99, 261, 287–89; access, 283; unsafe, 283

abuse: childhood, 117; sexual, 3, 165, 168, 303, 317, 319. *See also* violence: interpersonal

accessibility, 259, 303, 323, 326

adolescence, 65, 74, 80, 310, 317

advocacy, 114, 115, 324

African, 23, 264, 267, 270, 332

African American, 246

alcohol, 7, 10, 93, 146, 241, 235; abuse, 162, 181

American Samoa, 43, 44, 330, 332

anxiety, 3, 30, 51, 53, 76, 117, 118, 166, 286

apartheid, 188, 192, 194, 317, 318

avian flu, 1

Bangladesh, 210, 299, 300–301, 332

beliefs, traditional, 1, 74, 75, 76, 134, 162, 213, 225, 261, 271, 275–76, 324, 332

birth control, 65, 97, 114, 311–12, 323; access, 65; pill, 97, 323

bisexual, 52, 61, 66

Blackfeet, 167, 181, 182, 184, 207

body image, 51, 65

BRAC, 299–301, 303

Brazil, 52, 53, 59, 97, 291, 292, 296, 298, 325, 331; Amazon, 292, 325, 331

breastfeeding, 111, 113, 332

bullying, 29, 27, 118, 166, 167, 137

caregivers, 162, 228

caste, 41, 308

cervical cancer, 211, 246, 249–50, 320–23

charter school, 308–10

childhood, 60, 74, 96, 117, 120, 153, 168, 320

Christian, 266

chronic illness, 8, 9, 196, 259, 333

church, 3, 7, 48, 49, 108, 127, 136, 139, 238, 266, 269, 271, 273, 277

circumcision, 66, 67, 74, 75, 77–79

clinic, 36, 83, 84, 86, 96, 99, 100, 104, 139, 147, 161, 261, 263, 267, 269, 271, 273–76, 283, 289, 298, 300, 323, 326, 327; community, 259–60, 271–72; free, 168; health, 228, 260; rural, 46, 145, 213, 228, 229, 260; teen, 175

community
—action, 303, 304
—awareness, 4
—change, 47, 48, 207, 299
—collective, 2
—empowerment, 133, 303, 330
—gay, 51, 54, 59, 60
—health, 1, 3, 4, 161, 210, 211, 225, 255, 302–4; narratives, 5, 305; programming, 5; workers, 47, 48, 77, 291–92, 294, 299, 300, 323, 324–26
—intervention, 149, 299
—investment, 216
—leader of, 77, 78
—meetings, 219, 293
—members, 136, 156, 316, 326
—organizations, 244
—rural, 5, 101, 284, 291–92, 299–302, 324

community (*continued*)
—urban, 5, 10, 302
contraception, 65, 88, 97, 114–15, 311, 313, 323; emergency, 85
counselors, 16, 17, 62, 119, 161–62, 168
culture, 2, 5, 27, 53, 66, 74, 75, 77, 151, 196, 317, 325, 330; traditions, 66, 300
Cure Violence, 206–7, 303, 319

depression, 3, 117–19, 162, 166, 168, 210, 309, 314–16
Detroit, Michigan, 173, 174, 180, 300, 319
diabetes, type 2, 35, 37, 210, 333
disability, 261; learning, 162; long-term, 209; physical, 278; psychiatric/psychological, 120 (*see also* mental illness)
disease, 35, 45, 90, 117, 165, 166, 206, 209, 211, 212, 219, 224, 225, 227, 229, 230, 231, 233, 246, 255, 256, 260, 274, 307, 308, 310, 318, 323, 325; chronic, 210, 309; communicable (infectious), 1, 2, 3, 4, 7, 8, 196, 207, 209–11, 303; management, 8, 307; noncommunicable, 209, 210, 211; prevention, 209, 210, 256, 274, 321; treatment, 261; tropical, 3, 255, 256. *See also specific diseases*
drugs, 10, 11, 23, 26, 46, 127, 128, 131, 181, 196, 235
drunk driving, 184, 211, 244

education, 5, 8, 10, 65, 114, 115, 151, 161, 194, 200, 209, 211, 228, 235, 245, 284, 285, 303, 310, 325, 328

Facebook, 7, 24, 26, 27, 31–34, 47, 49, 150, 316
family: hardship, 255; member, 7, 8, 9, 37, 61, 101, 117, 118; support, 35, 307
female genital mutilation, 74
Florida, 27, 28, 31, 196, 197, 201, 331
friendship, 9, 33, 51, 80, 87, 156

gay, 51–55, 58–61, 63, 66, 83, 87, 303
Gay-Straight Alliance (GSA) Network, 61–63

gender, 4, 63, 65–67, 80, 85, 302, 303, 310, 329, 333; identity, 61, 63, 85
guinea worm disease, 211, 224, 233
gun violence. *See* violence: interpersonal

H1N1. *See* swine flu
Haiti, 119, 133, 134, 136, 203, 315
health care: access, 4, 259, 261, 262, 301, 303, 323–24, 334; affordability, 259, 260, 303, 323, 326; availability, 259, 260, 303, 323, 326; provider, 8, 67, 161, 228, 259, 261, 262, 283, 321, 325
health insurance, 118, 175, 250, 251, 260, 261, 327. *See also* health care: access, affordability
health problems, 2, 3, 4, 117, 118, 166, 196, 209, 246, 259, 260, 309, 314, 318; poor health outcomes, 181; due to poor nutrition, 43
HIV/AIDS, 18, 117, 162, 166, 169, 170, 188, 191, 196, 209, 267, 274, 307, 309, 318, 328, 329
homelessness, 130
human papillomavirus (HPV), 246, 249, 252, 255, 322–23
human trafficking, 196

illiteracy/illiterate, 275, 269, 299
imported, 40, 308
India, 35, 36, 119, 149, 150–54, 157, 161–62, 182, 186, 299, 302, 308, 330, 331, 333
inequality, 317, 318
infection, 74, 77, 87, 166, 206, 216, 225, 255, 256, 263, 274, 283, 288, 300, 318
internally displaced persons, 262, 266, 324
intervention, 1, 4, 9, 161, 210, 211, 261, 299, 303. *See also* community: intervention
Iraq war, 314

Johannesburg, South Africa, 188, 191, 194, 319

lesbian, 52, 61, 66
Lima, Peru, 284, 288
low-income countries, 210, 246

Maasai, 66, 74, 77–79
marijuana, 120, 126, 128
medical technology, 261, 278
mental health, 3, 5, 117–19, 161, 162, 165, 166, 167, 302, 313–14, 318, 330, 331, 332, 333
mental illness, 1, 2, 4, 17, 118, 119, 130, 131, 133, 161, 162, 302, 303, 313–16, 331. *See also specific illnesses*
Mexico, 226, 303, 329
Montana, 161, 182, 303

negative emotions, 3, 27, 149, 154, 155

overweight, 8, 30, 31, 34, 43, 51; obesity, 1, 43, 210

Pap smear, 246, 250, 285, 322
Peru, 261, 284, 285, 334
Planned Parenthood, 83
policy, health, 328, 330
post-traumatic stress disorder (PTSD), 3, 117, 119, 140, 145–46, 165, 314, 315, 329
poverty, 3, 10, 118, 165, 166–67, 181, 299, 303, 314; extreme, 181
pregnancy, 65, 67, 84, 85, 88, 101, 108, 114, 172, 216, 283, 289, 294, 310, 311, 312; prenatal care, 67, 99, 101; teen, 88, 95–99; unintended, 312
prevention, 4, 114, 209–12, 225, 255, 256, 302, 303, 310, 316, 320, 321; short-term, 210; sexually transmitted infections (STIs), 114, 310, 313; suicide, 316. *See also* disease: prevention
psychological trauma, 139, 145, 146, 147, 315
psychotic disorders, 120
puberty, 65, 67–68, 70, 72–73, 90, 310–13
public health, 24, 228, 261, 330; advocates, 114; global, 5; programs, 4; workers, 228

quality, 2, 10, 118, 161, 259–61, 303, 317, 318

rape, 165, 167, 266, 274, 317

refugee, 149, 150, 262, 263, 273, 275, 299, 323–24, 330
rehabilitation, 162
relationships, 3, 4, 7, 98, 246, 247, 322, 331, 333; negative, 7; romantic, 65; same-sex, 66; sexual, 65; social, 2, 8, 9, 51, 117, 118, 302. *See also* sexual; social support; social ties
religion, 131, 330
reproductive health, 180, 329; decisions, 302; policy, 328; problems, 246
reservation, 166, 181, 183, 207
resilience, 159, 330

Sabin Vaccine Institute, 255–56, 303
Sangath, 161–63, 303
sanitation, 3, 17, 320; systems, 210
schizophrenia, 117–20, 124–26, 162, 210
self-esteem, 7, 9, 27, 101, 118
sexual: education, 65, 114–15, 303; health, 65, 114, 313, 329, 334; initiation, 33, 310; orientation, 52, 61, 63, 65, 66, 80, 303; sexuality, 4, 53, 65, 67, 80, 101, 289, 302, 310, 313, 333. *See also* sexually transmitted infections
sexually transmitted infections (STIs), 65, 114, 210, 312, 322. *See also specific infections*
slum, 300
social conditions, 133, 165
social isolation, 180
social network, 7
social pressures, 133
social support, 8, 10, 101, 117, 118, 181, 308
social ties, 4, 7, 8, 9, 210, 307
South Africa, 164, 167, 207, 317, 318, 330, 331, 332
South Sudan, 212–13, 224, 303, 330
stigma, 101, 191, 313, 318
sub-Saharan Africa, 263
suicide, 118, 119, 127, 129, 130, 314, 316, 329
swine flu (H1N1), 211, 225–34

teacher, 10, 11, 12, 18, 19, 21, 23, 58, 61, 62, 90, 123, 142, 152, 168, 170, 173, 174, 198,

teacher (*continued*)
201, 202, 227, 228, 230, 242, 264, 267,
269, 272, 284, 305, 313, 314, 319
teenager, 52, 53, 60, 65, 67, 97, 101, 168, 188,
213, 244, 297, 313, 316, 331
Tibet, 149, 151–53, 158, 302
training, 61, 67, 132, 141, 149, 160–63, 260,
292, 297, 314, 333
transgender, 52, 61, 66
traumatic experiences, 3, 117, 119, 140, 165,
211, 243
Twitter, xii, 7, 316

Uganda, 262, 265, 266, 268, 272, 273, 330
unemployment, 165, 188
United States, 3, 5, 10, 35, 43, 67, 88, 118,
168, 181, 196, 203, 204, 205, 226, 233,
235, 236, 246, 256, 259, 260, 262, 263,
265, 272, 278, 302, 311, 314, 316, 326,
328, 329, 330, 331, 332, 334
urban, 5, 10, 167, 285, 300, 302

vaccines, 96, 212, 228, 229, 234, 255, 256
violence, 1, 3, 4, 52, 61, 151, 165, 166, 167,
181, 188, 191, 195, 196, 206, 207, 302,
303, 307, 318, 319, 320, 332; interpersonal, 1, 4, 117, 165, 167, 168, 188, 191,
196, 303, 317, 319; intertribal, 207;
political, 119, 149; structural, 165, 181,
196, 303, 317

World Health Organization (WHO), 2,
65, 74, 77